15⁵⁰

Advanced Life Support for the USMLE Step 2

Advanced Life Support for the USMLE Step 2

Matt Flynn
Ben Yeh
Lynn Anthony
Ketan R. Bulsara
Albert S.Y. Chang
Theresa McCarthy Flynn
Bryan J. Krol
Jay B. Rao

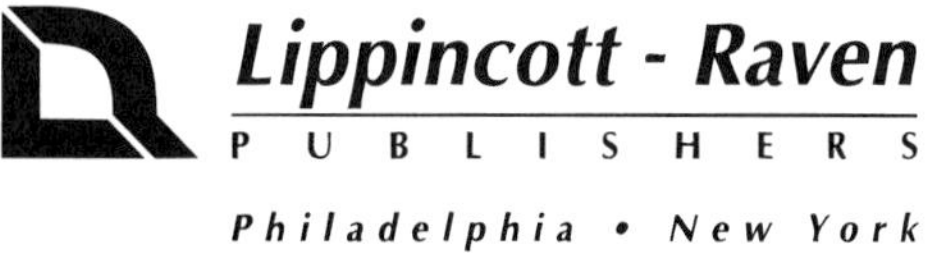
Lippincott - Raven
PUBLISHERS
Philadelphia • New York

Acquisitions Editor: Richard Winters
Developmental Editor: Mary Beth Murphy
Associate Managing Editor: Elizabeth A. Durand
Production Manager: Caren Erlichman
Production Coordinator: MaryClare Malady
Design Coordinator: Melissa Olson
Indexer: Lynne Mahan
Compositor: Maryland Composition Company, Inc.
Printer: Maple Press

Library of Congress Cataloging-in-Publication Data

Advanced life support for the USMLE step 2 / Matt Flynn . . . [et al.].
p. cm.
Includes index.
ISBN 0-397-58436-9 (pbk. : alk. paper)
1. Medicine—Outlines, syllabi, etc. I. Flynn, Matt.
[DNLM: 1. Medicine—outlines. 2. Licensure, Medical—outlines.
WB 18.2 A244 1997]
R834.5.A38 1997
610′.76—dc20
DNLM/DLC
for Library of Congress 96-41668
CIP

Care has been taken to confirm the accuracy of the information presented and to describe generally accepted practices. However, the authors, editors, and publisher are not responsible for errors or omissions or for any consequences from application of the information in this book and make no warranty, express or implied, with respect to the contents of the publication.

The authors, editors, and publisher have exerted every effort to ensure that drug selection and dosage set forth in this text are in accordance with current recommendations and practice at the time of publication. However, in view of ongoing research, changes in government regulations, and the constant flow of information relating to drug therapy and drug reactions, the reader is urged to check the package insert for each drug for any change in indications and dosage and for added warnings and precautions. This is particularly important when the recommended agent is a new or infrequently employed drug.

Some drugs and medical devices presented in this publication have Food and Drug Administration (FDA) clearance for limited use in restricted research settings. It is the responsibility of the health care provider to ascertain the FDA status of each drug or device planned for use in their clinical practice.

9 8 7 6 5 4 3 2 1

Contributors

Matt Flynn
Department of Internal Medicine
University of California at San Francisco
San Francisco, California

Ben Yeh
Department of Radiology
University of California at San Francisco
San Francisco, California

Lynn Anthony
Department of Radiology
North Carolina Baptist Hospital
Bowman Gray School of Medicine
Winston-Salem, North Carolina

Ketan R. Bulsara
Division of Neurosurgery
Duke University Medical Center
Durham, North Carolina

Albert S. Y. Chang
Department of Surgery
Baylor College of Medicine
Houston, Texas

Theresa McCarthy Flynn
Department of Pediatrics
University of California at San Francisco
San Francisco, California

Bryan J. Krol
Department of Otolaryngology—Head and Neck Surgery
Indiana University Medical Center
Indianapolis, Indiana

Jay B. Rao
Duke University Law School Class of 1998
Durham, North Carolina

All of the authors were members of the Duke University School of Medicine class of 1996.

Preface

The United States Medical Licensing Exams are a time-consuming and expensive part of becoming a doctor licensed to practice in the United States. Over the past few decades, hundreds of books of varying quality have been written to help students pass the exams. Nevertheless, in our studies we found no good review of that small but critical set of facts that get tested again and again.

Advanced Life Support is a guide to the most heavily tested facts on the USMLE Step 2. The book was written by medical students immediately after taking the exam. The point of *Advanced Life Support* is to get you the most points for your studying time. During the editing process, all the fluff was mercilessly cut out. Each chapter was then carefully reviewed for accuracy by at least two experts in the relevant field.

We recommend first reviewing the introduction and the study hints provided at the beginning of each chapter. You may also want to skim the book to get a better feel for what is important. As the exam date draws near, spend some time mastering the chapters to make sure that you are not giving away easy points.

Best of luck on the exam!

Acknowledgments

Each chapter in *Advanced Life Support for the USMLE Step 2* was carefully reviewed for accuracy by top clinicians in that field. Many thanks are due to the following individuals for their patience and excellent advice on improving the manuscript.

Barbara Sheline, MD

Robert Reed, MD

Karen Perkins, MD

Alex Kemper, MD

Caroline Haynes, MD, PhD

Marvin Hage, MD

Melissa Garretson, MD

Eric M. Gabriel, MD

John Dimaio, MD

Michael Cuffe, MD

Jose E. Cavazos, MD, PhD

Murray Abramson, MD

Thanks for the inspiration are also due to the authors of *Crashing the Boards: A Friendly Study Guide for the USMLE Step 1*, in particular Joseph Paydarfar, Shankha Biswas, Sean Wu, and Lawrence Liao.

Contents

Advanced Life Support for the USMLE Step 2, by Flynn et al.
Lippincott–Raven Publishers © 1997.

CHAPTER 1

The USMLE Step 2

First, the good news. The USMLE Step 2 is more interesting, more relevant, and just plain more pleasant than the USMLE Step 1. If you have taken the USMLE Step 1, the worst is over. If you haven't, you have our heartfelt sympathies.

The bad news is that just like Step 1, the USMLE Step 2 covers an enormous amount of material. Harrison's and Cecil's combined don't answer all of the internal medicine questions, and there are several other fields.

Fortunately, one can do very well on the test by mastering a much smaller, well-selected set of information. *Advanced Life Support* was written by medical students immediately after taking the USMLE Step 2. It is a concise review of the most heavily tested facts designed to maximize your score by making sure you get the easy points.

We have paid particular attention to important topics that students tend to overlook. Smoking cessation, dermatology, fractures, and medicolegal issues are all good examples of heavily tested subjects that you may not have had much exposure to. We also cover important facts from more familiar topics. At every step, we took great care to ensure that only the most valuable information made it into print.

What the USMLE Step 2 Really Tests

The USMLE Step 2 is a test of clinical knowledge. Unlike the USMLE Step 1, almost all Step 2 questions are directly relevant to the practice of medicine. The main subject areas are internal medicine, obstetrics and gynecology, pediatrics, psychiatry, preventive medicine, and surgery. There are also questions on legal and social issues. Internal medicine is perhaps the most tested subject due to its sheer size. It is followed by obstetrics and gynecology, psychiatry, and pediatrics in no particular order.

The USMLE Step 2 emphasizes outpatient medicine. Preventive medicine, risk factor interventions, and common outpatient problems come up repeatedly. Tertiary hospital inpatient care is not emphasized, even though it comprises the majority of rotation time for most U.S. medical students.

The USMLE Step 2 also emphasizes emergency medicine. A large number of the surgery questions in particular deal with emergencies such as trauma and the acute abdomen. Many more questions address urgent and emergent problems from the other major fields.

Relatively few questions ask for a diagnosis. Questions are more likely to ask for the best treatment option, the next lab test to order, or the best preventive measure. The test is made harder by several questions that give a classic disease description, then ask about etiology or epidemiology without naming the disease. In addition, **the best answer may not be on the list of options.**

The Basics of the Board Exams

The United States Medical Licensing Examinations are required for certification. To be licensed to practice medicine in the United States, a physician must pass all three steps. The first two steps are traditionally taken before beginning internship. The third step is usually taken during residency. With few exceptions, Board certification in a field requires passage of all three USMLE exams, completion of an accredited residency, and passage of field-specific exams.

The USMLE Step 2 is given over two days. There are two 3-hour sessions each day, with one test booklet per session. An examinee must break the seals on all four test booklets for his or her exam to be scored.

Early registration is required. A passport photo, application form, and check payable in U.S. dollars on a U.S. bank must be received approximately **three months** before the exam.

Each test booklet contains a variable number of questions, typically 171 or 181. The last question asks whether you had enough time to complete the test. The USMLE Step 2 employs the same three types of questions used in the USMLE Step 1. Question types are grouped together to minimize errors based on misunderstanding instructions. The first 120 to 140 questions are in the one-best-answer format. Each question has four or five options. The next few questions use the EXCEPT format. Test instructions will make it clear when the EXCEPT questions begin. The final section gives lists of 4 to 26 answers with one or more associated questions. The Step 2 answer sheet often has more than the relevant number of bubbles. If there are eight options, there may be anywhere from 8 to 26 bubbles.

The last test booklet, given during the afternoon of the second day, contains about 60 high-quality photographs. X-rays, dermatology, retinal disease, and other photogenic subjects are emphasized in the last booklet.

Making Your Studying Count

You will probably have less time to study for the USMLE Step 2 than for Step 1. Many students take rotations right up to exam day and do not have the luxury of devoting a month to preparing for the exam. Step 2 does take most students less time to prepare for, but there are still several key subjects that should be learned well. **Use the study hints at the beginning of each chapter to guide your efforts.**

Talk to people who have taken the exam to get a feel for the test. Don't believe people who say the exam is easy. The USMLE Step 2 is considered easier than Step 1, primarily because the material tends to be more familiar. Nevertheless, Step 2 is still quite hard, and it appears to be getting harder and longer.

Probably the most critical point is to **study what you do not know.** Do not spend a lot of time studying the finer points of your best subject areas. If you are good at internal medicine, study other subjects first, or at least concentrate on those topics in internal medicine that are less familiar to you.

Start by studying a topic area you like but do not know well. Many students enjoy obstetrics or pediatrics, for example, but have not retained enough from their introductory rotations. You will learn the material better and faster if it is interesting to you. Later you can knuckle down to study the more boring subjects.

As always, you should study when your brain is working. If you are an evening person, study in the evening. If circumstances force you to study at a bad time, enlist the help of friends, coffee, or whatever works for you.

Study material that is concise and memorable. If you used a good short text for the course, then by all means reread it if you have time. Most importantly, use whatever you will actually read.

Use active learning to your advantage. Quiz yourself periodically, and try to recall facts from memory. Many students find question books useful for this purpose. Question books can be very effective, but be advised that **the questions in question-format review books are generally much shorter than those on the exam.**

Finally, you may notice some theme topics during the first day. If you feel up to it, look up the answers to some of the theme questions you didn't know. Don't spend too much time on it.

Test-Taking Strategies

- Make sure you answer all questions. **There is no penalty for guessing.**
- **Time is the enemy.** The questions are *long*. As you start each booklet, note the number of questions. It varies, but is usually 171 or 181. Time yourself page-by-page if you don't happen to be the world's fastest test taker. Many students find it useful to spend the first 30 seconds writing

out a timeline. If the test starts at 1:05 p.m., then write on the inside cover:

Time	*Questions Finished*
1:35	30
2:05	60
2:35	90
3:05	120
3:35	150
4:05	End of exam

Timelines are especially useful on the first test booklet because many students do not finish it. Keep in mind that the timeline represents the slowest pace that will complete the booklet.

- At least one test preparation course advises reading each question twice. Avoid doing that whenever possible. There is not time.
- The first few questions can be quite flustering. Keep moving!
- Do the questions in order on the page.
- Fill in your answers in batches. A good batch size is one page (about 6–10 questions). This will save time and reduce errors.
- It may be faster to do the matching lists first.
- Check your answer if you have time.
- There will be a few absurd questions on the exam. Some are experimental; others are just very detailed. For example, a case may present a child with the signs and symptoms of Kawasaki's disease, then ask what treatment will prevent long-term sequelae. Shrug your shoulders, choose your favorite letter, and move on. Check the question at the end to make sure you didn't miss something obvious. Don't let them get you down.

Avoiding Stupid Errors and Overcoming Ignorance

- Read each question carefully. We're not kidding. People tend to get lazy about reading questions as the exam wears on. If you miss the word "not," you get the question wrong.

- For long clinical scenarios, read the last sentence first. The last sentence usually contains the question. You will save time by knowing what to look for as you read.
- For matching lists, make sure you read the introductory sentence—e.g., "For each of the following causes of chest pain, . . ." As you read the cases that follow, keep in mind that chest pain (or whatever) is the hallmark symptom.
- Go with your initial choice unless you have a *good* reason for switching.
- When asked to choose a number, choose one of the middle two answers if you are not sure.
- In match lists, answers are rarely correct twice. When in doubt, do not repeat an answer.
- Be wary of choosing tertiary interventions. Often the point is to avoid doing anything drastic. When in doubt, choose the minor treatment or the available variant of CLOMI (Cat-Like Observation and Masterful Inactivity).
- Surgery patients are a different story. For them, tertiary is good.
- **Do not despair if all the questions seem hard.** Like the USMLE Step 1, the average score on the USMLE Step 2 is somewhere around 65%. On most tests, that is a flunking grade. In other words, you should expect to do far worse on the USMLE Step 2 percentage-wise than you have on almost every other test you have taken.

Comfort Measures

The day before the exam, you'll want to gather everything you'll need for test day. Make sure you have your admission ticket, a valid photo I.D., and directions to the test center. You may also want a jacket, watch, earplugs, analgesia, caffeine, a couple of #2 pencils (optional), and perhaps some food. Test conditions vary. The air conditioning may be locked on, or you may not be able to see the clock. Rest assured that the exam will proceed regardless of what happens.

The morning of the exam, keep in mind that your bladder is not your friend. You will be allowed to go to the bathroom one at a time and with an escort. No extra time will be given, even if you drank two double espressos. On the same note, don't eat a big lunch . . . sleeping is not good.

Best of luck on the exam!

Advanced Life Support for the USMLE Step 2, by Flynn et al.
Lippincott–Raven Publishers © 1997.

CHAPTER 2

Preventive Medicine

*Theresa McCarthy Flynn
and Lynn Anthony*

Study Hints

- Preventive medicine is short but very high yield.
- Several questions ask for the single most effective intervention for a given disease.
- Smoking cessation is high yield.
- Cancer screening schedules are high yield.
- Contraindications to specific vaccines are high yield.
- Memorizing childhood immunization schedules is low yield. Recommendations vary from year to year and state to state, and past exams have provided a schedule.

Pregnancy

- **Folate** prevents **open spinal cord defects** such as spina bifida.
- **Iron** prevents maternal anemia.

Infancy and Childhood

- The leading cause of infant mortality in the U.S. is **congenital anomalies.**

- **Infant mortality** is the number of deaths of *liveborn* infants before the first birthday per 1000 live births.
- Effective prevention measures include **immunizations,** proper use of **car seats,** and **fluoride** to prevent dental caries.

NEWBORN SCREENING

All states screen newborns for disorders that benefit greatly from early intervention.

- **Phenylketonuria** (PKU) is an autosomal recessive disorder in which phenylalanine hydroxylase activity is reduced. Toxic metabolites cause severe **mental retardation.** PKU test results are not accurate if blood is drawn in the first 24 hours of life. If an initial PKU test is positive, **repeat the test** first to confirm the diagnosis. **Restrict dietary phenylalanine by age 3 weeks** to prevent mental retardation.
- Galactosemia is an autosomal recessive disorder in which galactose-1-phosphate uridyltransferase activity is reduced. Liver failure, renal tubular dysfunction, and **cataracts** develop when the infant ingests the galactose in **milk.** Death may follow. **Avoid all milk,** including breast milk, to prevent disease. Special formulas are required.
- Maple syrup urine disease is an autosomal recessive deficiency of the decarboxylase that degrades the branched chain amino acids leucine, isoleucine, and valine. Infants die without treatment. Treat by **restricting branched-chain amino acids.**
- Hypothyroidism results in cretinism if it is not treated. The newborn screen measures T4 levels. If a newborn tests hypothyroid, **get another T4 level** to confirm disease and **check a TSH** to determine if the hypothyroidism is primary or secondary. Treat with thyroid hormone.

Young Adults

- The leading cause of death in the United States from **age 1 to 44** is **accidents.** Motor vehicle accidents account for half of these deaths.

- Half of motor vehicle accident deaths involve **alcohol use** by one or both drivers. **Minimum drinking age laws** reduce mortality from motor vehicle accidents.
- The leading cause of death in the United States of **men aged 25 to 44** is **AIDS.**

Adulthood

- Overall, the leading causes of death in the United States are **heart disease,** then **cancer,** then **stroke.**
- Several questions will describe adults with one or more health problems, then ask for the single most effective intervention. If there is one disease, treat according to the table below. For patients with multiple diseases, **smoking cessation** is often the best choice.

DISEASE PREVENTION

Disease	*Single Best Preventive Measure*
Heart disease	**Stop smoking.**
Stroke	Treat **hypertension,** including isolated systolic hypertension.
Colon cancer	Eat adequate fiber.
Osteoporosis	Give postmenopausal estrogen therapy.

BENEFITS OF SMOKING CESSATION

Time After Stopping	*Benefits*
Immediate	**Peptic ulcer healing improved**
	Lung symptoms reduced (cough, phlegm production)
1st trimester of pregnancy	Risk of low birth weight eliminated
	Mental retardation reduced

Time After Stopping	*Benefits*
Years	**MI risk decreased to non-smoker levels in 2–4 years**
	Lung cancer reduced up to 90%
	Risk of oral, esophageal, pancreatic, and bladder cancer reduced to non-smoker levels
	Risk of stroke reduced
Other effects	**No reversal of COPD**
	Average **weight gain of 5 pounds**

- About 80% of ex-smokers relapse within a year.

MANAGEMENT OF HIGH CHOLESTEROL

Lab Finding	*Action*
Total cholesterol <**200**	Repeat in 5 years
Total cholesterol 200–239 without other risk factors	Diet and repeat in a year
Total cholesterol >**240** ***or*** >**200 with two risk factors**	**Check LDL**
LDL cholesterol >160 *or* >130 with two risk factors	Diet
LDL cholesterol >190 *or* >160 with two risk factors	Drugs
LDL cholesterol >130 with **coronary** disease	Drugs with **goal LDL <100**

- Risk factors include male sex, family history of coronary artery disease before 60 years of age, smoking, hypertension, severe obesity, diabetes mellitus, low HDL, hyperlipidemia, and definite cerebrovascular disease or peripheral vascular disease.
- **The first-line drug treatment is cholestyramine** (a bile-acid binding resin).
- HMG-CoA reductase inhibitors (lovastatin, simvastatin, pravastatin) are the most effective drugs.

- Weight loss in the obese reduces cholesterol, blood pressure, blood glucose, and triglycerides.

ESTROGEN REPLACEMENT THERAPY

- Postmenopausal estrogen **reduces cardiovascular deaths and hip fractures** in women.
- It may **increase the risk of breast cancer.**
- The risk of **endometrial cancer** is increased only if estrogen is given without progesterone. Naturally, if the woman does not have a uterus, endometrial cancer is not a consideration.
- Overall, postmenopausal estrogen decreases mortality.
- Estrogen replacement therapy also prevents vaginal atrophy.
- Smoking is not a contraindication to postmenopausal estrogen.

DIABETES MANAGEMENT

- **Good glucose control** slows the progression of **diabetic retinopathy** and **renal disease.**
- **ACE inhibitors** help prevent the progression of **renal insufficiency.**
- **Well-fitting shoes** help prevent diabetic foot injury.
- Pregnant diabetics need very tight control of glucose levels.

CANCER

- **Lung cancer** is the leading cause of cancer death in both sexes.
- Breast cancer is the #2 cause of female cancer death. It is the leading cause of cancer death in women who do not smoke.
- Prostate cancer is the #2 cause of male cancer death. It is the leading cause of cancer death in men who do not smoke.
- Colorectal cancer is the #3 cause of cancer death in both men and women, making it the #2 cause of cancer death overall.

CANCER SCREENING

Cancer	*Screening Test*	*Frequency*	*Starting Age*
Colorectal	Stool occult blood	Yearly	50
	Sigmoidoscopy	**q2 years,** then q3–5 years	**50**
Cervical	Pap smear/ pelvic exam	Yearly	18 or first coitus
Breast	Physician exam	Yearly	40 or 50
	Mammography	Baseline and q1–2 years	**40**

- There is controversy about breast cancer screening schedules. At this time, the American Cancer Society, American Medical Association, and American College of Obstetrics and Gynecology recommend mammography every 1–2 years between the ages of 40 and 69. Other groups recommend baseline mammograms at age 50.

Immunizations

CHILDHOOD IMMUNIZATIONS

- The Sabin oral polio vaccine (OPV) contains a live virus that is shed in feces for several weeks. **Do not give live OPV to infants living with an immunocompromised person.** Give the *k*illed Sal*k* vaccine instead.
- Most bad reactions to DPT are caused by the **pertussis** component. Give *a*ttenuated pertussis vaccine (D*a*TP) to infants who react to their initial DPT vaccine.
- **The exam will probably provide immunization schedules if needed.**

SAMPLE SCHEDULE

	Birth	*2 mos*	*4 mos*	*6 mos*	*1 yr*	*15 mos*	*5 yrs*	*12 yrs*
Hep B	X	X		X				
DPT		X	X	X	X		X	
OPV		X	X	X	X		X	
HIB		X	X	X	X			
MMR						X		X

HepB, hepatitis B; *DPT,* diphtheria, pertussis, tetanus; *OPV,* oral polio vaccine; *HIB, Hemophilus influenzae* B; *MMR,* measles, mumps, rubella.

ADULT IMMUNIZATIONS

- Give a **single** pneumococcus vaccination to patients with **asplenia,** chronic heart or lung disease, or diabetes.
- Give **annual** influenza virus vaccinations to health care workers, people over age 65, and patients with chronic disease. Never give influenza, measles, or mumps vaccines to anyone with a severe **egg allergy.**
- Give Td (tetanus and *low dose* diphtheria) vaccinations **every 10 years.** Adults do not get pertussis vaccine.

PREGNANCY

- **Do not give MMR** (measles, mumps, rubella) or the Sabin live polio vaccine to pregnant women. Live virus vaccines are not given in pregnancy.

Legal Issues

RIGHT TO REFUSE CARE

- **The right to refuse care takes precedence over all other legal considerations.**
- Do not force Jehovah's Witnesses to accept blood products.

RIGHT TO INFORMED CONSENT

- Informed consent must be obtained for any **diagnostic procedure, intervention, or therapy.** Patients have the **right to change their minds at any time.**
- The patient must receive an **explanation** of the procedure or therapy, its purpose, and the **risks and side effects.** The patient should then be allowed to ask any questions. Consent must be given before the process can begin.
- Informed consent is **not needed for emergency care,** treatment of sexually transmitted diseases, or treatment of specific reportable diseases such as tuberculosis.

HEALTH CARE DECISIONS

- A **health care power of attorney** allows a designated representative to make health care decisions in the event a patient becomes incompetent.
- **Living wills** direct health care decisions in **specific** medical situations. "Do Not Resuscitate" directives are one example. Living wills do not mean automatic DNR status.
- In the absence of clear patient wishes, a health care power of attorney, or an applicable living will, health care decisions are made for the patient **by close family members with the treating or primary care physician.**

PARENTAL CONSENT LAWS

- Minors have the right to **substance abuse treatment** and **medical care during pregnancy** without parental consent. In many states, minors also have the right to treatment of sexually transmitted diseases without parental consent.

GOVERNMENT PROVISIONS

- **Medicaid** is government health insurance for the **poor.**
- **Medicare** is government health insurance for people >**65 years old,** disabled individuals who are entitled to Social Security benefits, and end-stage renal disease patients. It covers inpatient care, home health visits, and 100 days of posthospitalization care in a skilled nursing facility. **Medicare does not pay for long-term care.**

Statistics

OVERVIEW

- Sensitivity, specificity, and predictive value are measures of how good screening tests are. Each has an important and unique role to play.

	Has Disease	***No Disease***
Positive test	a	b
Negative test	c	d

- Sensitivity $= \frac{a}{a + c}$.
- Specificity $= \frac{d}{b + d}$.
- Odds ratio $= \frac{ad}{bc}$. Odds ratios are used for **retrospective** studies.

SENSITIVITY

- **Sensitivity is the proportion of people with a disease who test positive for the disease.**
- High sensitivity tests **detect everyone who has the disease.** In other words, there are **few false negatives.** High sensitivity says nothing about the number of false positives.
- Good screening tests usually have high sensitivity.

SPECIFICITY

- Specificity is the proportion of people *without* a disease who test negative for the disease.
- High specificity means **false positives are rare,** so a positive result is reliable. High specificity tests **verify disease.**
- High specificity says nothing about the number of false negatives. A negative result does not rule out disease unless the test also has high sensitivity (Fig. 2-1).

PREDICTIVE VALUE

- Predictive values answer the question, "How likely is it that my test result is accurate?"
- **Positive predictive value** is the proportion of people who test positive who do indeed have the disease. It is **true pos-**

Sensitivity Versus Specificity

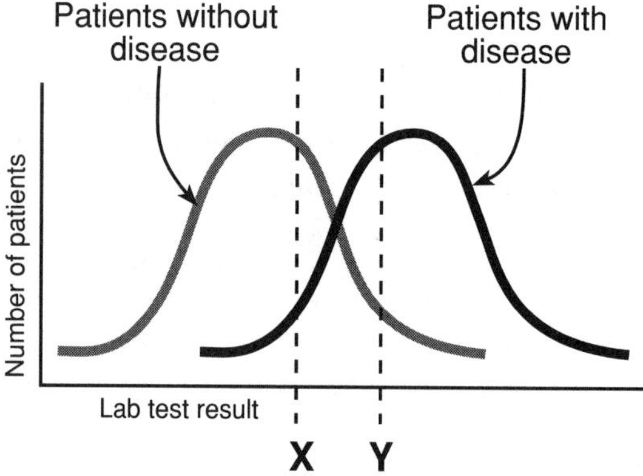
Patients without disease
Patients with disease
Number of patients
Lab test result
X
Y

General points

- **X** and **Y** are two different values of a lab test to be used by a hospital as a cutoff point for the normal range.
- **Choosing X creates a highly sensitive test** (few false negatives). The test will have low specificity because there will be many false positives.
- **Choosing Y creates a highly specific test** (few false positives). The test will have low sensitivity because there will be many false negatives.
- **Sensitivity and specificity are not mutually exclusive**. A given test may be both sensitive and specific, only one and not the other, or neither.

Figure 2-1

itives divided by **all positives.** True positives are persons who test positive for a disease *and* actually have the disease.

- **Positive predictive value is highest when the disease prevalence is high.** A 60-year-old woman with a positive mammogram is more likely to have breast cancer than a 40-year-old woman with a positive mammogram. Put another way, 60-year-old women have more true positive tests, so the ratio of true positives to all positives is higher.
- Negative predictive value is true negatives divided by all negatives.
- **Negative predictive value is highest when the disease prevalence is *low*.**

POPULATION STATISTICS

- **Incidence** is the number of **new** cases in a given time period, usually a year.

- Prevalence is the number of cases (old and new) present **at a single moment in time.**
- The 1-year incidence exceeds the prevalence for short-term illness—e.g., the incidence of flu may be 1.2 million cases in a given year, while the prevalence on any given day is <100,000 cases.
- Prevalence exceeds incidence for long-term illnesses. There are more diabetics at any given time than there are new cases of diabetes diagnosed in a year.

Advanced Life Support for the USMLE Step 2, by Flynn et al.
Lippincott–Raven Publishers © 1997.

CHAPTER 3

Psychiatry

Jay B. Rao

Study Hints

- Several questions ask you to distinguish psychopathology from normal reactions (e.g., depression versus normal grief).
- The diagnosis and treatment of common problems such as depression, anxiety, and substance abuse are high yield.
- Schizophrenia is high yield.
- Child psychiatry is high yield.
- Psychotropic drugs and their side effects are high yield.
- Do *not* memorize DSM-IV criteria.

Psychotic Disorders

- Psychosis is **an inability to distinguish what is real from what is not.**
- Prominent features include hallucinations, delusions, and disorganized thought.
- Most psychotic disorders are treated with antipsychotic drugs such as **haloperidol** (Haldol).
- Psychosis can be caused by medications and ''nonpsychiatric'' diseases.

SCHIZOPHRENIA

- Schizophrenia is **equally common in men and women,** but appears earlier in men. There are no racial differences.
- The lifetime prevalence is 1–1.5%.
- Risk factors include **birth in the winter, birth hypoxia,** and a positive family history.
- **Psychosis** is a hallmark.
- Positive symptoms include hallucinations, delusions, loose associations, and bizarre behavior. Treat positive symptoms with **antipsychotics.**
- Negative symptoms include social withdrawal, blunted affect, poverty of speech, and catatonia. Treat refractory negative symptoms with **clozapine** or risperidone.
- The diagnosis requires **6 months** of symptoms.
- **Premorbid level of functioning** is the most useful prognostic sign.
- Excess dopaminergic activity is a proposed mechanism.
- Suicide is a major risk.

OTHER PSYCHOTIC DISORDERS

- **Brief psychotic disorder** is the presence of psychosis for **at least 1 day but less than 1 month.** It is brought on by marked stress. Hospitalization and treatment with antipsychotics and benzodiazepines are often required.
- **Schizophreniform disorder** refers to schizophrenia symptoms that last between **1 and 6 months.** If it lasts longer than 6 months, it is schizophrenia.
- **Delusional disorder** involves **non-bizarre delusions** (such as being followed) that last more than 1 month. Hallucinations consistent with the delusion may be present. Treat with antipsychotics.

Substance Abuse (Fig. 3-1)

- Abuse means at least **1 month** of impairment leading to negative consequences.
- Dependence means abuse for more than 6 months accom-

Drug Abuse

Cocaine

- Cocaine causes **euphoria followed by depression**.
- Physical signs include mydriasis, hypertension, and tachycardia.
- Use can lead to **cardiac arrhythmias** and **psychosis**.
- Treat psychosis with **haloperidol** (Haldol). Treat severe hypertension and hyperthermia with **phentolamine**.
- Withdrawal may cause **cravings**, hypersomnolence, and depression.
- Give **tricyclic antidepressants** (desipramine) to reduce cravings.

Alcohol

- Alcohol abuse is very common, especially among **men**. 13% of people abuse alcohol.
- Intoxication causes disinhibition, poor judgment, CNS depression, and ataxia.
- **Overdose can lead to coma and death**.
- Treat dependence with **group therapy** and possibly disulfuram or naltrexone.
- Withdrawal may cause **delirium tremens** (DTs) and seizures.
- **Prevent and treat DTs with benzodiazepines**.

Phencyclidine (PCP)

- PCP is a hallucinogen that causes **violent behavior**, clouded sensorium, fantasies, and euphoria.
- Physical signs include mydriasis and nystagmus.
- **PCP can cause seizures and coma.**
- Treat violent behavior with haloperidol. Treat seizures with benzodiazepines.

Barbiturates

- **Women** and people from **upper socioeconomic classes** most commonly abuse barbiturates.
- Intoxication causes **sedation**, **analgesia**, and **euphoria**.
- Physical signs include **miosis**, hypotension, and diaphoresis.
- Use can lead to **blunted respiratory drive, coma**, and seizures.
- Treat overdose with **emesis**, **gastric lavage**, and **urine alkalinization**. Use hemodialysis and life support as necessary.
- Withdrawal can be fatal.

Opioids

- Heroin abuse is three times more common in **men**. The typical age of onset is in the **30's**.
- Heroin's effects include **sedation**, **euphoria**, and **hypoactivity**.
- Physical signs include **needle track marks**, **miosis**, decreased respiratory drive, and flushed warm skin.
- **Shock, coma, pulmonary edema**, and hypotension may be present.
- Treat overdose with **supportive care** and **naloxone** (Narcan).
- Withdrawal may cause cravings, mydriasis, sweating, abdominal pain, and "gooseflesh" (piloerection).
- Wean addicts with **methadone**. Prevent withdrawal symptoms with **clonidine**.

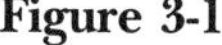

Figure 3-1

panied by drug-seeking behavior, failed attempts to quit, and withdrawal symptoms.

Mood Disorders

- Mood is an individual's internal emotional condition.
- Affect is the external expression of mood. A person can be depressed (depressed mood) but appear normal (normal affect).

DEPRESSION

- **Unmarried people and women** are most at risk for depression.
- There are **no racial differences** in the incidence of depression.
- The mean age of onset is 40.
- The lifetime prevalence of depression is 15%.
- Symptoms include DESPAIR, feelings of worthlessness, and guilt.
    - **D**epressed mood
    - **E**nergy loss
    - **S**uicidal ideation or attempts
    - **P**sychomotor retardation or agitation
    - **A**nhedonia
    - **I**nsomnia or hypersomnia
    - **R**educed appetite or increased appetite
- Treat depression with **selective serotonin reuptake inhibitors** (SSRIs) such as fluoxetine (Prozac). Tricyclic antidepressants (TCAs) and Wellbutrin may also be used.
- Electroconvulsive therapy (ECT) is normally reserved for refractory disease.
- Treatment reduces the average duration of symptoms from 6–12 months to 3 months.
- **Low serotonin activity** is one proposed etiology. Most antidepressants increase serotonin levels.

- **Atypical depression** is characterized by **hyperphagia** and **hypersomnolence.** Treat with **monoamine oxidase inhibitors** (MAOIs).
- Postpartum depression is characterized by depression and thoughts of harming self or the child. Treat with antidepressants.
- Be able to distinguish depression from normal grief. Brief intense longing is normal even years after the loss of a loved one.

DEPRESSION VERSUS GRIEF

Depression	*Normal Grief*
Suicidality	No suicidality
Feelings of worthlessness; self blame	**Feelings of loss;** crying
Occasional psychotic symptoms	No psychotic symptoms
Lasting functional impairment	Return to emotional baseline within 1 year

BIPOLAR DISORDER

- Unmarried people and those from higher socioeconomic classes are most at risk.
- There are **no racial or gender differences.**
- The mean age of onset is 30.
- The lifetime prevalence is 1%.
- **Elevated, expansive, or irritable mood** is the hallmark. **Pressured speech, flight of ideas,** grandiosity, impulsivity, and mood-congruent delusions may be present.
- Often patients will have a history of multiple speeding tickets, sexual promiscuity, or outrageous buying sprees.
- Treat mania with one of the mood stabilizers **lithium, valproate,** or carbamazepine. You should not be asked to choose between lithium and valproic acid (valproate). If you are, the question is old and you should choose lithium.

- Continual prophylaxis with lithium is indicated after two episodes of mania.
- Treat depression with antidepressants.

SUICIDE

- Suicidal intent is a psychiatric emergency. Patients with suicidal ideation or plans must be hospitalized, against their will if necessary.
- Women are more likely to attempt suicide. Men are more likely to succeed.
- Caucasians, unmarried people, and those with a family history of suicide are most at risk.

Anxiety Disorders

- Anxiety is **the experience of fear in the absence of a real threat.**
- Treat with behavioral therapy, psychotherapy, cognitive therapy, and benzodiazepines.

PANIC DISORDER

- **Women** are twice as likely to have panic disorder. It usually appears in young adulthood.
- **Intense anxiety accompanied by dyspnea, chest pain, palpitations, and dizziness** is characteristic. Attacks usually last about 30 minutes. They can mimic heart attacks.
- **Agoraphobia,** or the irrational fear of leaving home, is linked to panic disorder.
- Treat with imipramine (a TCA), SSRIs, or benzodiazepines. Systematic desensitization and cognitive therapy may be helpful.

PHOBIAS

- A phobia is an irrational fear of an object or situation that leads to avoidant behavior.
- Treat with behavioral therapy and systematic desensitization. β-blockers reduce the autonomic manifestations of fear.

OBSESSIVE COMPULSIVE DISORDER

- Obsessive compulsive disorder is characterized by recurrent thoughts (obsessions) and repetitive ritualistic actions (compulsions) that impair functioning. Common obsessions include thoughts of violence, worrying that the stove is on, and worrying that the doors are unlocked. Common compulsions include repeated showering and repeated handwashing.
- Patients recognize that their obsessions and compulsions are abnormal.
- Treat with **clomipramine,** SSRIs, and behavioral therapy. On older test questions clomipramine may not be an option, in which case you should choose the SSRI.
- **Serotonin** may be involved. Clomipramine and SSRIs block serotonin uptake.

Somatoform and Related Disorders

BODY DYSMORPHISM

- Body dysmorphic disorder is characterized by **preoccupation with an imagined defect** in the body. Diagnose it only when the preoccupation is not better explained by anorexia nervosa or some other somatoform disorder.

HYPOCHONDRIASIS

- Hypochondriasis is the chronic fear that one has a serious illness despite a lack of medical evidence.
- Treat with regularly scheduled short appointments.

SOMATIZATION

- Somatization disorder is characterized by multiple somatic complaints without an identifiable physical cause.

CONVERSION

- Conversion disorder is characterized by sudden **neurologic symptoms** that have no identifiable physical cause. Numb hands and feet are classic.

- Patients are relatively unconcerned about the dysfunction **("la belle indifference").**

SOMATOFORM PAIN DISORDER

- Somatoform pain disorder is characterized by pain without an identifiable physical cause.

FACTITIOUS DISORDER AND MALINGERING

- In both factitious disorder and malingering, the patient has **voluntary control of physical symptoms.**
- In factitious disorder, **the motive is unconscious.** In other words, the behavior is deliberate, but the reason for choosing the behavior is not clear to the patient.
- Malingering is not a mental disorder. It is characterized by conscious and deliberate faking of illness with a **conscious motive.**

Personality Disorders

- Personality disorders are diagnosed only when personality traits become maladaptive and impair social functioning.
- Treat cluster A disorders with antipsychotics and psychotherapy.
- Treat all other personality disorders with psychotherapy.

Cluster A (Odd, Eccentric)	*Characteristics*
Paranoid	Unwarranted suspicion and mistrust; blames others
Schizotypal	Odd beliefs, behavior, appearance, and thinking (positive symptoms of schizophrenia without psychosis)
Schizoid	**Social withdrawal;** indifference to others; prefers isolation

Cluster B (Emotional, Erratic)	*Characteristics*
Antisocial	Disregard for others; criminality; aggression; co-morbid substance abuse; childhood history of torturing animals and setting fires; no proven treatment
Borderline	Unstable mood; self-mutilation; suicide attempts; typically loves or hates a person, often both in the same day
Histrionic	Dramatic behavior; flamboyant dress; more prevalent in women
Narcissistic	Sense of entitlement; grandiosity; lack of empathy

Cluster C (Anxious, Fearful)	*Characteristics*
Avoidant	**Fear of criticism** or rejection; social withdrawal; inferiority complex; **dislike their isolation** (versus schizoid people)
Dependent	Lets others assume responsibility; fear of abandonment
Obsessive-compulsive	Preoccupied with order, rules, and details; rigid and stubborn

Psychopharmacology

SIDE EFFECTS

Problem	*Drug(s) of Choice*	*Side Effects*
Depression	SSRIs	Few side effects
	TCAs	Overdose fatal; anticholinergic effects such as dry mouth, blurred vision, constipation, and sedation

Problem	*Drug(s) of Choice*	*Side Effects*
	MAO-Is	**Hypertensive crisis** with tyramine-rich foods such as cheese and beer; orthostasis; anticholinergic effects
Mania	Lithium	**Hypothyroidism;** tremor; renal dysfunction
Psychosis	Neuroleptics	Parkinsonism; tardive dyskinesia; acute dystonia; **neuroleptic malignant syndrome** (all with high-potency neuroleptics); anticholinergic effects (with low-potency neuroleptics)
Anxiety	Benzodiazepines	Sedation; tolerance; dependence
	Buspirone	No sedation; no tolerance; no abuse; no withdrawal

- Tardive dyskinesia involves involuntary movements such as lip smacking and sucking.
- Acute dystonic reaction is an idiosyncratic focal muscle spasm, such as torticollis, which appears hours or days after starting a high-potency neuroleptic like haloperidol.
- Neuroleptic malignant syndrome is a rare life-threatening side effect of antipsychotics. Symptoms and signs include rigidity, fever, organ failure, and elevated creatine phosphokinase (CPK).

Child Psychiatry

TOURETTE'S SYNDROME

- Tourette's syndrome is characterized by **motor tics** and **vocal tics.** Motor tics are involuntary, purposeless motor movements. Vocal tics include involuntary swearing.

- Patients are typically boys aged 7–8.
- Treat tics with **haloperidol.**

ADHD

- Attention deficit hyperactivity disorder (ADHD) is characterized by a shortened attention span, difficulty concentrating, increased motor activity, and impulsivity.
- ADHD is much more common in **boys.**
- Treat with stimulants such as **methylphenidate** (Ritalin).

OPPOSITION VERSUS CONDUCT

- Children with oppositional defiant disorder (ODD) argue with adults, **lose their temper,** and **blame others** for their own misbehavior. They do *not* typically torture animals, destroy property, or steal. Social and academic problems are common. Symptoms typically begin by age 8 and not later than adolescence. Treat with behavioral therapy.
- Conduct disorder is the childhood version of antisocial personality disorder. Conduct disorder is characterized by **aggression** against people and animals and an **inability to follow societal norms.** Affected kids often repeatedly **destroy property, lie, or steal.**
- Evidence of conduct disorder during childhood is required for the diagnosis of antisocial personality disorder in an adult.

ELIMINATION DISORDERS

- Encopresis is fecal incontinence. It is pathological only after age 5. It occurs more commonly in boys. Medical illnesses such as Hirschsprung's disease must be ruled out first. Treatment includes **family therapy.**
- Enuresis is bedwetting. **It is pathological only after age 5.** Genitourinary anomalies and other medical conditions must be ruled out. Treat with appropriate toilet training and behavior therapy. **Imipramine** is rarely used anymore except for refractory cases, but the Boards still ask about it. Choose imipramine only if all of the other options are drugs.

SEPARATION ANXIETY DISORDER

- Separation anxiety *disorder* is most common in **7- to 8-year-olds.**
- Symptoms must last for at least **4 weeks.** They include excessive distress when separated from mom or another major attachment figure, nightmares about separation, and physical symptoms such as headaches or stomach cramps when separation occurs.
- **School avoidance is a hallmark.**
- Treat with psychotherapy and imipramine.

Eating Disorders

ANOREXIA NERVOSA

- **Adolescent women** from wealthy families are most at risk. Patients are typically good students.
- The hallmarks are **a decrease in body weight more than 15% below normal** and a refusal to maintain normal body weight. Other signs and symptoms include abnormal feelings about food, a disturbed body image, excessive exercise, and laxative abuse.
- **Amenorrhea** may be the presenting symptom.
- Treat initially with supervised feedings and family and individual psychotherapy. Cyproheptadine is also used.
- Anorexia nervosa can be fatal. Hospitalize if necessary.

BULIMIA NERVOSA

- Age of onset is either adolescence or early adulthood.
- Patients are usually at or near **normal body weight.** Weight fluctuations are typical.
- **Menstruation is normal.**
- Patients binge on food, then purge by vomiting or by using laxatives.
- Fingernail changes and throat abrasions are common in patients who induce vomiting.
- Treat with **SSRIs,** individual psychotherapy, and behavioral therapy.

Adjustment Disorders and Grief

ADJUSTMENT DISORDERS

- These disorders represent maladaptive responses to stressful life events such as death or divorce.
- They are more common in women and hospitalized patients.
- Symptoms include **excessive stress** or other mood disturbance with significant **impairment of functioning.**
- Symptoms develop within 3 months of a stressful event and resolve within 6 months.
- Treat with **psychotherapy.**

NORMAL GRIEF

- Normal grief can involve intense feelings of loss, crying spells, depressed mood, and a decreased enjoyment of life.
- Dysfunction may occur, but it is not overwhelming or lasting.
- Adjustment disorders are diagnosed when dysfunction becomes pronounced or lasting.

Delirium Versus Dementia

Delirium	*Dementia*
Altered consciousness	Impaired cognition with **normal consciousness**
Caused by toxins, systemic disease	Caused by degeneration, as with Alzheimer's
Rapid onset	Slow onset
Symptoms fluctuate	Symptoms stable
Usually **reversible**	Usually irreversible
Treat underlying cause	Symptomatic treatment
Common in intensive care units	Common in the elderly and nursing home residents

Advanced Life Support for the USMLE Step 2, by Flynn et al.
Lippincott–Raven Publishers © 1997.

CHAPTER 4

Pediatrics

Lynn Anthony
and Theresa McCarthy Flynn

Study Hints

- Age is often the most important clue to diagnosis in pediatrics.
- Questions involving children may not be testing pediatrics. Kids get appendicitis.
- Infectious diseases such as epiglottitis that are specific to pediatrics are high yield.
- Genetic syndromes are high yield.
- Routine care of children is high yield. Questions focus on developmental issues and prevention.
- Pediatric fractures are high yield. They are discussed in the chapter on the glossy book (Chapter 9).

Development

DEVELOPMENTAL MILESTONES

Figure 4-1 illustrates some developmental milestones.

Developmental Milestones

Newborn

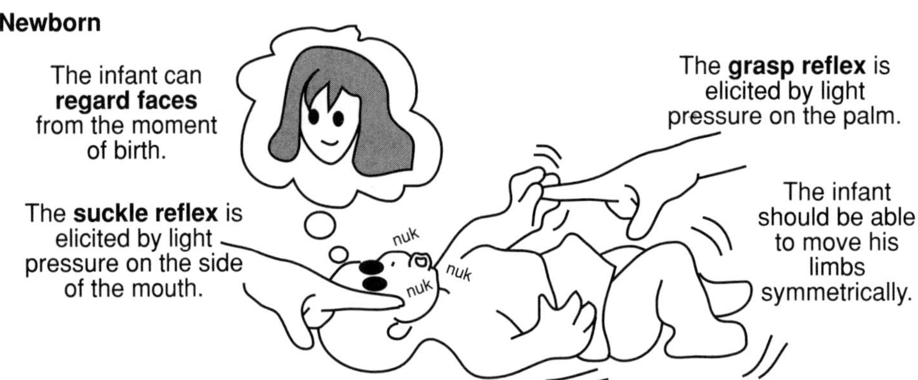
The infant can **regard faces** from the moment of birth.
The **grasp reflex** is elicited by light pressure on the palm.
The **suckle reflex** is elicited by light pressure on the side of the mouth.
nuk
nuk
nuk
The infant should be able to move his limbs symmetrically.

The **Moro reflex** causes the arms and legs to extend, then flex, when the head is suddenly extended.

Social smile @ 4-6 wks

Six months

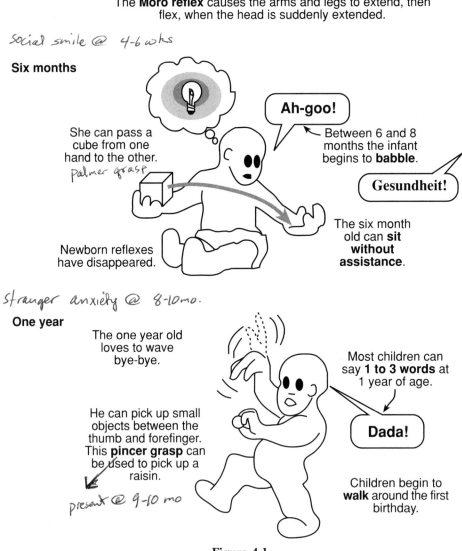

She can pass a cube from one hand to the other.

palmer grasp

Ah-goo!

Between 6 and 8 months the infant begins to **babble**.

Gesundheit!

The six month old can **sit without assistance**.

Newborn reflexes have disappeared.

Stranger anxiety @ 8-10 mo.

One year

The one year old loves to wave bye-bye.

Most children can say **1 to 3 words** at 1 year of age.

Dada!

He can pick up small objects between the thumb and forefinger. This **pincer grasp** can be used to pick up a raisin.

present @ 9-10 mo

Children begin to **walk** around the first birthday.

Figure 4-1

Two years

The two-year-old uses **2-to 3-word phrases**.

Go up!

She can build a tower of 4 blocks.

Two-year-olds have learned how to climb up steps.

Three years

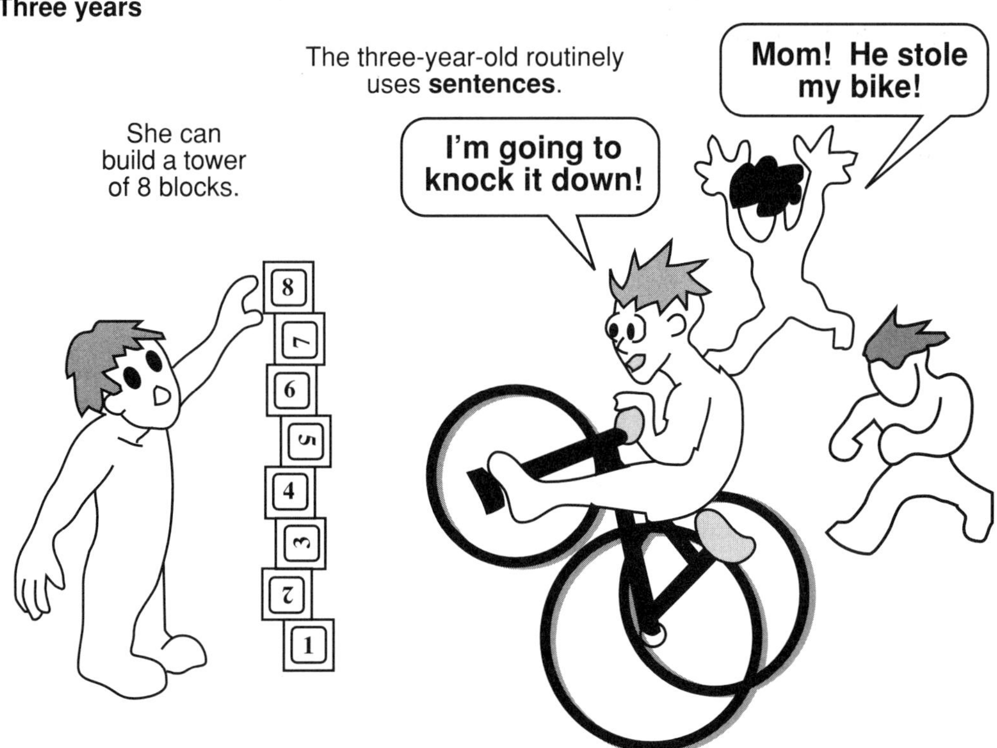
The three-year-old routinely uses **sentences**.
Mom! He stole my bike!
She can build a tower of 8 blocks.
I'm going to knock it down!
8
7
6
5
4
3
2
1

The three-year-old can ride a tricycle and begins to play interactive games such as tag.

DEVELOPMENTAL ANXIETIES

- Stranger anxiety appears at 7–9 months. The infant has a tendency to cry and cling to mom when a stranger appears.
- Separation anxiety peaks at 18 months.

Infectious Disease

STREPTOCOCCAL INFECTIONS

- The #1 cause of neonatal sepsis and meningitis is **Group B *Streptococcus.*** (*B*abies get Group *B.*) *E. coli* is the #2 cause of serious neonatal infection.
- Group A *Streptococcus (Streptococcus pyogenes)* causes pharyngitis, impetigo, and **scarlet fever.** Scarlet fever typically presents with a red punctate rash 24–48 hours after pharyngitis first appears.
- Poststreptococcal glomerulonephritis is most common after **treated** Group A *Strep* **skin infections. Nephritic syndrome** (hematuria, hypertension, and edema) with evidence of previous *Strep* infection is diagnostic. Treat with diuretics and antihypertensives. About 95% of patients recover completely.
- Rheumatic fever is most common after **untreated** Group A *Strep* **pharyngitis.** A mnemonic for the major Jones criteria is JONES:

  J Joints (migratory arthritis)
  ♡ Carditis
  N Nodes (subcutaneous nodes)
  E Erythema marginatum
  S Sydenham's chorea
- Treat rheumatic fever with **aspirin** to reduce inflammation and **lifetime prophylactic penicillin** to prevent endocarditis. **Mitral valve stenosis** is the most common valve complication.

MENINGITIS

Age of Onset	*Most Common Organism*
<2 mo	**Group B *Streptococcus***
2 mo to 6 y	*Streptococcus pneumoniae*
7 y and older	***Neisseria meningitidis***

- *Streptococcus pneumoniae* replaced *Hemophilus influenzae* as the #1 cause of bacterial meningitis sometime around 1991 thanks to the HIB vaccine. The Boards may not have caught up. However, you should not choose *H. influenzae* unless *Strep pneumoniae* is not an option.
- You *should* choose ***H. influenzae*** as the #1 cause of **epiglottitis.** There is no longer any clear #1 cause of epiglottitis. If the question is asked, it is an old question.

REYE SYNDROME

- Reye syndrome involves encephalopathy and liver failure in children and adolescents.
- Influenza and varicella viruses are most strongly associated with Reye syndrome.
- For Boards purposes, **aspirin** is not given to children with viral infections because it is thought to cause Reye syndrome. The evidence is weak.

CONGENITAL INFECTIONS

- The mnemonic is **TORCH.**
- Clinical features of TORCH infections include intrauterine growth retardation, nonimmune hydrops fetalis, anemia, and jaundice.
- ***T*oxoplasmosis** is caused by a parasite in cat feces. It can manifest as a ring-enhancing brain lesion.
- **"*O*ther"** includes varicella zoster, syphilis, HIV, and hepatitis B.
- ***R*ubella** is dangerous in the first trimester. It causes patent ductus arteriosus, congenital deafness, and varying degrees of mental retardation.
- ***C*ytomegalovirus** produces a distinct petechial rash ("blueberry muffin rash") in addition to the features common to most TORCH infections.
- ***H*erpes simplex** can be transmitted during vaginal delivery if the mother has active lesions. Mothers with active genital herpes should be delivered by cesarean section.

Respiratory Disease in Infants and Children (Fig. 4-2)

RESPIRATORY DISTRESS SYNDROME (Fig. 4-2)

- **Surfactant deficiency** causes RDS in **preterm infants.**
- A **ground glass appearance** on chest x-ray is characteristic.
- Patients may have a **patent ductus arteriosus.**
- Treat with surfactant and supportive care.
- **Oxygen** is usually required but often causes **bronchopulmonary dysplasia** and **blindness due to retinopathy of prematurity.**

Gastrointestinal Disease in Children

(Fig. 4-3)

Genetic Disease

PEDIGREE ANALYSIS

- Autosomal dominant diseases usually appear in every generation.
- X-linked recessive defects are seen mainly in male offspring and can skip generations.

GENETIC PROBABILITIES

- The odds of a child with one heterozygous parent inheriting an autosomal dominant trait are 50%.
- The odds of a child with two carrier (heterozygous) parents inheriting an autosomal recessive trait are 25%.
- If a mother is carrying an X-linked recessive trait, 50% of male children will be affected and 50% of female children will be carriers.

Respiratory Distress in Infants and Children

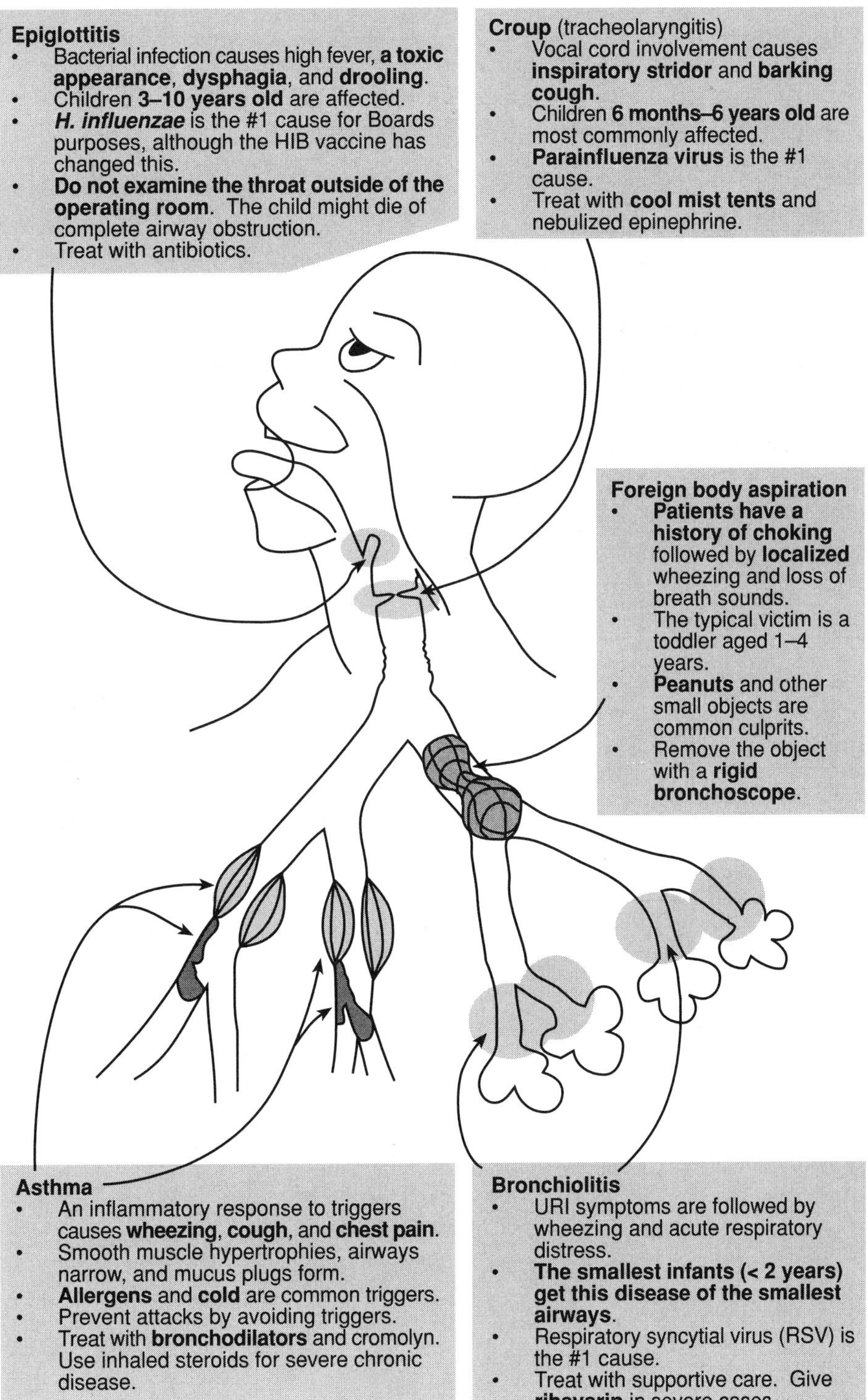

Epiglottitis
• Bacterial infection causes high fever, **a toxic appearance**, **dysphagia**, and **drooling**.
• Children **3–10 years old** are affected.
• ***H. influenzae*** is the #1 cause for Boards purposes, although the HIB vaccine has changed this.
• **Do not examine the throat outside of the operating room**. The child might die of complete airway obstruction.
• Treat with antibiotics.
Croup (tracheolaryngitis)
• Vocal cord involvement causes **inspiratory stridor** and **barking cough**.
• Children **6 months–6 years old** are most commonly affected.
• **Parainfluenza virus** is the #1 cause.
• Treat with **cool mist tents** and nebulized epinephrine.
Foreign body aspiration
• **Patients have a history of choking** followed by **localized** wheezing and loss of breath sounds.
• The typical victim is a toddler aged 1–4 years.
• **Peanuts** and other small objects are common culprits.
• Remove the object with a **rigid bronchoscope**.
Asthma
• An inflammatory response to triggers causes **wheezing**, **cough**, and **chest pain**.
• Smooth muscle hypertrophies, airways narrow, and mucus plugs form.
• **Allergens** and **cold** are common triggers.
• Prevent attacks by avoiding triggers.
• Treat with **bronchodilators** and cromolyn. Use inhaled steroids for severe chronic disease.
Bronchiolitis
• URI symptoms are followed by wheezing and acute respiratory distress.
• **The smallest infants (< 2 years) get this disease of the smallest airways**.
• Respiratory syncytial virus (RSV) is the #1 cause.
• Treat with supportive care. Give **ribavarin** in severe cases.

Figure 4-2

Gastrointestinal Disease in Children

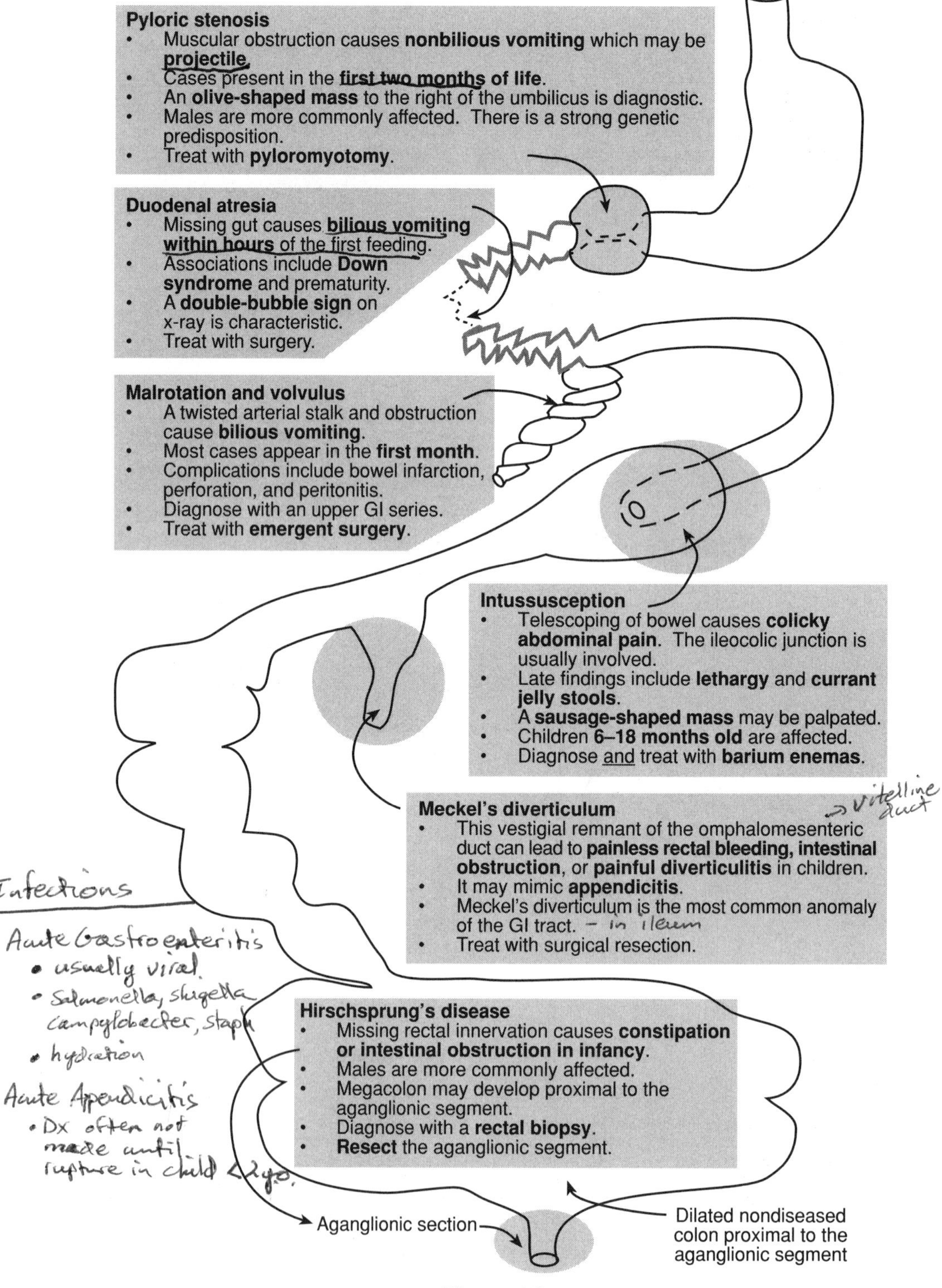

Pyloric stenosis
• Muscular obstruction causes nonbilious vomiting which may be projectile.
• Cases present in the first two months of life.
• An olive-shaped mass to the right of the umbilicus is diagnostic.
• Males are more commonly affected. There is a strong genetic predisposition.
• Treat with pyloromyotomy.
Duodenal atresia
• Missing gut causes bilious vomiting within hours of the first feeding.
• Associations include Down syndrome and prematurity.
• A double-bubble sign on x-ray is characteristic.
• Treat with surgery.
Malrotation and volvulus
• A twisted arterial stalk and obstruction cause bilious vomiting.
• Most cases appear in the first month.
• Complications include bowel infarction, perforation, and peritonitis.
• Diagnose with an upper GI series.
• Treat with emergent surgery.
Intussusception
• Telescoping of bowel causes colicky abdominal pain. The ileocolic junction is usually involved.
• Late findings include lethargy and currant jelly stools.
• A sausage-shaped mass may be palpated.
• Children 6–18 months old are affected.
• Diagnose and treat with barium enemas.
Meckel's diverticulum
→ vitelline duct
• This vestigial remnant of the omphalomesenteric duct can lead to painless rectal bleeding, intestinal obstruction, or painful diverticulitis in children.
• It may mimic appendicitis.
• Meckel's diverticulum is the most common anomaly of the GI tract. – in ileum
• Treat with surgical resection.
Infections
Acute Gastroenteritis
• usually viral
• Salmonella, shigella campylobacter, staph
• hydration
Acute Appendicitis
• Dx often not made until rupture in child <2yo.
Hirschsprung's disease
• Missing rectal innervation causes constipation or intestinal obstruction in infancy.
• Males are more commonly affected.
• Megacolon may develop proximal to the aganglionic segment.
• Diagnose with a rectal biopsy.
• Resect the aganglionic segment.
Aganglionic section
Dilated nondiseased colon proximal to the aganglionic segment

Figure 4-3

CYSTIC FIBROSIS

- **Chloride ion channels** are defective in cystic fibrosis. A **sweat test** will reveal increased chloride in sweat.
- **Bronchiectasis** (dilated, damaged bronchi), hemoptysis, and ***Pseudomonas*** pneumonia are common.
- Gastrointestinal manifestations include **meconium ileus** and **pancreatitis.**
- Patients with pancreatic insufficiency require pancreatic enzymes and the fat soluble vitamins A, D, E, and K.

DOWN SYNDROME

- Down syndrome (trisomy 21) occurs in 1 in 800 live births. Incidence increases with the age of the mother.
- The #1 cause is **maternal nondysjunction.**
- Features include mental retardation, congenital heart disease, palmar creases, and small jaws.
- Down children have an increased risk of **duodenal atresia, leukemia,** and **Alzheimer's disease.**
- If you are given a karyotype, look for trisomy 21.

TURNER SYNDROME

- Patients are 45,XO females.
- **Mosaicism** may be responsible for the variable severity of the disease.
- Clinical features include **webbed neck,** short stature, shield chest with widely spaced nipples, and **regression of ovaries to fatty streaks.**
- **Bicuspid aortic valves** and **coarctation of the aorta** are relatively common in Turner patients.

KLINEFELTER SYNDROME

- Patients are 47,XXY males.
- The incidence increases with maternal age.
- Clinical features include hypogonadism, infertility, long limbs, mild mental retardation, and gynecomastia.
- Treat by giving testosterone at the time of puberty.

47,XYY MALES

- These males demonstrate increased **aggression** and represent a relatively high proportion of prison populations.

PRADER-WILLI SYNDROME

- Prader-Willi syndrome results from a defect or deletion in the **paternal** chromosome 15.
- It leads to **obesity,** small genitals, severe hypotonia, and failure to thrive.

21-HYDROXYLASE DEFICIENCY

- This defect prevents production of cortisol and aldosterone. All precursors are shunted to the androgen synthesis pathway.
- Clinical features include **ambiguous genitalia in females** and **salt-wasting** in either sex.
- Cortisol, aldosterone, and urine 17-hydrocorticosteroids are decreased. **Urine 17-ketosteroids** are increased.
- Treat with **hydrocortisone** titrated to avoid the development of Cushingoid features, **mineralocorticoids** for salt-wasting infants, and **NaCl** supplementation in the first year of life.
- Complications include **premature epiphyseal fusion** from excess androgens and death.

Hematology

ERYTHROBLASTOSIS FETALIS

- Erythroblastosis fetalis, or hemolytic disease of the newborn, is caused by blood group incompatibility between mother and fetus. The mother produces IgG against antigens on fetal red blood cells.
- Affected mothers most commonly have **Rh negative** blood and are carrying an Rh positive fetus. The risk of disease increases when fetal blood crosses into the maternal circulation.
- Events that increase exposure to fetal blood include first-trimester abortion, ectopic pregnancy, amniocentesis, and motor vehicle accidents.

hemolysis is extravascular

- Neonates present with anemia, hyperbilirubinemia, hepatosplenomegaly, pulmonary edema, and ascites.
- The **direct Coombs test** will be positive.
- Treat with supportive blood transfusions. *CHF, resp. distress, acidosis, + hypotension are risks of HgB too low*
- Prevention is possible with **Rhogam** (anti-Rh IgG) injections for high-risk mothers at 28 weeks, at delivery, and at any other time of exposure to fetal blood.
- *Can cause hydrops fetalis - in utero*

NEONATAL JAUNDICE

Initial Evaluation
- *CBC c̄ smear + Retic.*
- *Maternal + fetal blood types*
- *Coomb's test*
- *T & D [Bili]*

levels higher ~~seen earlier~~ + last longer in premies + last ≈ 7d

- **Physiologic jaundice** presents on days 3–4 of life with a serum bilirubin <20 mg/dL.
- Jaundice at birth indicates disease.
- Hemolytic jaundice is caused primarily by **blood-group incompatibility** or **sepsis.**
- The most serious complication of jaundice is **kernicterus.** In kernicterus, bilirubin deposits in brain cells, particularly in the **basal ganglia.**
- Symptoms of kernicterus include **seizures,** lethargy, hypotonia, and bulging fontanels.
- Treat jaundice with **phototherapy,** vigorous hydration, and exchange transfusion (if necessary).

SICKLE CELL ANEMIA

if s̄p CVA then @ high risk for recurrent + need reg. transfusion to HbS <30%

- In the United States, 8% of blacks are carriers.
- The defect is a point mutation that results in a valine substitution for glutamine in position 6 of the β-globin gene.
- Sickling is promoted by increased hemoglobin S concentration, fever, and acidosis.
- **Autosplenectomy** is common, resulting in an increased susceptibility to infection by encapsulated organisms. Patients need **pneumococcal and meningococcal vaccines.** Children <5 years get continual prophylactic penicillin.
- Watch for sickled cells on peripheral smears.
- *Vaso occlusive episodes - Analgesis, O₂ ~~PRBCs~~ PRBC's if hydration inadequate*

THROMBOCYTOPENIA

- Idiopathic thrombocytopenic purpura (ITP) manifests as low platelet count following an acute viral infection. It is usually self-limited. *1% mortality*
- *Bleeding of skin + mucous membranes c̄ severe bleeding after trauma*

- Avoid platelet transfusions in ITP unless active bleeding is present.
- Corticosteroids controversial
 - Refractory cases: IV gamma globulin, splenectomy or immunosuppressive agents

Oncology

LEUKEMIA

- Overall they are the #1 peds malignancy
- Risk factors:
 - Chromosome abnormalities
 - Immunodeficiency states
 - Identical Twins
 - SP Tx for solid tumor
 - congenital marrow failure
 - Schwachmann-Diamond
 - Diamond-Blackfan

- **Acute lymphoblastic leukemia** (ALL) is the #1 childhood cancer.
- Symptoms stem from **bone marrow failure** or from **extra-medullary involvement** such as CNS infiltration. Anemia, Hemorrhagic diathesis, Intxn, lymphadenopathy, Bone Pain
- Blood counts may be normal.
- Bone marrow biopsy is diagnostic.
- Treat with chemotherapy and **CNS irradiation. Allopurinol** is used during chemotherapy to reduce hyperuricemia. rapidly fatal s̄ Tx + often curable c̄ Tx
- Acute myeloblastic leukemia (AML) is distinguished from ALL by cell surface antigens and by the presence of **Auer rods** in leukemic cells. AML has a worse prognosis than ALL.

LYMPHOMA

differ from adult ← NHL
1) Predominantly extanodal presentation
2) T or B cell = frequency
3) Highly aggressive

Retinoblastoma - rare
- presents @ white reflex in the pupil
- Rb gene Ch. #13
- ↑ osteosarcoma + other malig. as adults
- Tx - surg. enucleation ± chemo

- All forms of lymphoma occur more often in boys.
- **Non-Hodgkin's lymphoma** (NHL) is more common in childhood.
    - **T-cell lymphomas** classically arise in the **anterior mediastinum** and may cause superior vena cava syndrome or pleural effusion.
    - **B-cell lymphomas** often arise in the gut, leading to **GI obstruction** or **intussusception.** Pain, ascites, urinary Tract obstrxn
    - Staging laparotomies are not done for pediatric patients.
    - All children with NHL receive systemic therapy because metastases are common. often outcome is favorable
- **Hodgkin's disease** usually involves the supraclavicular and cervical lymph nodes first. Constitutional symptoms are common.
    - **Reed-Sternberg cells** are pathognomonic for Hodgkin's disease. Lg., Binucleate cells c̄ inclusion like nucleoli

Staging

90% cure → I - one set of nodes

II - >1 node but on one side of diaphragm

III - Both sides of diaphragm

IV - extranodal - liver, bone, lungs

↗ 50% cure

- **Anergy** leads to increased risk of infections.
- Treat with **radiation** with or without chemotherapy.
- Prognosis for children is good.
- Treated patients often get secondary cancers years later. hypothyroidism, growth disturbances, sterility

CNS CANCERS

→ Medulloblastoma

- Most childhood primary brain tumors are **infratentorial.**
- **Increased intracranial pressure** may lead to headaches, vomiting, diplopia, or seizures.
- Treat with corticosteroids followed by surgery and irradiation.
- Brain stem gliomas usually not resectable
 - Astrocytomas have the best prognosis

WILMS TUMOR

- Wilms tumor classically presents with fever, abdominal pain, hematuria, and a flank mass.
- Polycythemia is a rare paraneoplastic complication.
- Patients younger than 2 years do much better.
- Treat with surgery plus radiation therapy.

- 2nd most common solid tumor of Childhood
- Mets common @ Diagnosis

Histiocytosis X
- proliferation of cells of reticuloendothelial system in periphery
- 3 syndromes
 Letterer-Siwe
 Hand-Schuller-Christian
 Eosinophilic granuloma

NEUROBLASTOMA

- **Neuroblastoma is the most common malignant tumor in infants less than 1 year old.**
- Cancer arises from **primitive neural crest cells** of the adrenal medulla or the sympathetic nervous system.
- Almost 50% of these tumors present as a hard, smooth, nontender flank mass.
- **Intravenous pyelograms** can help distinguish neuroblastomas from Wilms tumors. Neuroblastomas tend to displace the kidney without distortion of the calyces.
- Most neuroblastomas secrete one or more **catecholamines.**
- Treat with surgery and chemotherapy.
- Abdominal tumors have a worse prognosis than neuroblastomas found elsewhere.
- Patients less than 1 year old have the best prognosis.
- Head & Neck tumors present as palpable mass
 ± Horner's syndrome
 ↳ Miosis
 Ptosis
 Enophthalmos
 Anhidrosis

Noncyanotic Congenital Heart Defects

- Obstructive lesions and **left-to-right shunts** are noncyanotic.
- Presentations range from asymptomatic to severe congestive heart failure (CHF).
- CHF in children presents as failure to thrive, increased heart and respiratory rate, and dyspnea.

VENTRICULAR SEPTAL DEFECT

- **VSD is the most common congenital heart defect.**
- A pansystolic murmur at the left sternal edge is classic.
- Many small VSDs close spontaneously.
- Treat larger VSDs with medical management of congestive heart failure and antibiotic prophylaxis for endocarditis. Surgical repair should be performed before pulmonary hypertension develops.

ATRIAL SEPTAL DEFECT

- **Ostium secundum** defects are the most common *symptomatic* ASDs.
- Exam may reveal **a fixed and widely split S2.**
- Hemodynamically significant lesions are repaired surgically after the first year of life.

ATRIOVENTRICULAR SEPTAL DEFECT

- **Down syndrome** children account for most AVSDs.
- Patients present with congestive heart failure and first-degree heart block.
- Echocardiography is the diagnostic study of choice.
- Delay surgery until at least 3 months of age.

PATENT DUCTUS ARTERIOSUS

- **Prematurity** accounts for most cases of PDA. Congenital rubella is another cause.
- Exam reveals a **continuous machine-like murmur,** bounding pulses, and a wide pulse pressure.

- Close the ductus with **indomethacin** or surgical ligation *unless* the PDA is necessary for life due to another coexisting heart defect like transposition.

COARCTATION OF THE AORTA

- Patients often present in adulthood with delayed pulses and decreased blood pressure in the lower extremities.
- Chest x-rays classically show **rib notching** as a late finding.
- Associations include **bicuspid aortic valve** and **Turner syndrome.**

Cyanotic Congenital Heart Defects

- **All are right-to-left shunts.**
- **All require surgery.**

failure to thrive, tachypnea, cyanosis in 1st wks – months of life

TETRALOGY OF FALLOT

- **Tetralogy is the most common *cyanotic* congenital heart defect.**
- The tetralogy is right ventricular outflow tract obstruction, right ventricular hypertrophy, a ventricular septal defect, and an overriding aorta that opens onto both ventricles.
- **Tet spells** consist of sudden cyanosis, dyspnea, and mental status changes. Kids will squat to relieve their discomfort.
- Exam reveals a systolic murmur.
- Chest x-ray shows a **boot-shaped heart.**

TRANSPOSITION OF THE GREAT VESSELS

- Patients need a shunt such as an ASD, VSD, or PDA to survive.
- Three treatment steps exist. **Prostaglandin E_1** will keep a PDA open. **Balloon atrial septostomy** increases atrial mixing. **Surgically switching the atria or arteries** corrects the defect.

TRUNCUS ARTERIOSUS

- A single vessel replaces the aorta and the pulmonary artery. VSD will be present.
- Chest x-ray shows a **boot-shaped heart** with no distinct pulmonary artery.
- Treat by surgically defining a pulmonary artery and shunting right ventricular outflow to it.

ANOMALOUS PULMONARY VENOUS RETURN

- In this condition, some or all of the pulmonary venous return flows into the right heart.
- Total anomalous return is incompatible with life unless an ASD is present.
- Mild forms may present with increased frequency of pulmonary infections.

Neonatal Syndromes of Substance Abuse

ALCOHOL ABUSE

- The diagnosis of **fetal alcohol syndrome** requires **growth retardation** (<10th percentile), **characteristic facies** (microcephaly and underdeveloped midface structures), *and* **CNS symptoms** such as hypotonia, poor suck reflex, hyperactivity, or mental retardation.

TOBACCO ABUSE

- Tobacco use during pregnancy increases the risk of spontaneous abortion, premature delivery, and low birth weight.
- Affected children are more likely to suffer from **sudden infant death syndrome (SIDS),** developmental delays, and behavior disorders.
- No major structural anomalies have been associated with tobacco abuse during pregnancy.

COCAINE ABUSE

- Cocaine causes **vascular disruptions,** which can lead to several problems including placental abruption, spontaneous abortion, and congenital heart defects.
- Problems after the neonatal period include increased risk of sudden infant death syndrome, poor social behavior, and inappropriate response to environmental stimuli.

HEROIN ABUSE

- **Neonatal withdrawal syndrome** occurs within the first 24 hours of life.
- **High-pitched crying, fist sucking, food craving behavior, and tremulousness** characteristically appear early. Without treatment, hypotonia or seizures may occur.
- These children are typically small at birth but become normal in size.

Other Commonly Tested Disorders

NEPHROTIC SYNDROME

- Nephrotic syndrome is characterized by **massive proteinuria (>3.5 g/day), hypoproteinemia, hyperlipidemia, and edema.**
- **Lipoid nephrosis** (minimal change disease) is the most common cause of nephrotic syndrome in children. Treat lipoid nephrosis with **steroids.** Prognosis is good.
- Membranous nephropathy is the most common primary cause in adults. The disease results from immune complex deposition. There is no treatment available. Spontaneous remissions occur in 20%.
- Nephritic syndrome is a completely different disease entity characterized by hematuria, hypertension, and edema.

Rheumatic fever

- Complication of β-hemolytic strep infections
- Chorea found in children > adults

Tanner Staging

	♀	♂
I	preadolescent; Ø pubic hair →	
II	sparse hair along medial labia; breast & papilla slightly elevated	scant, long pubic hair; slight enlargement of penis & scrotum
III	↑'d dark pubic hair - begins to curl; breast & areola are enlarged	small amt of darker curlier hair; longer penis & larger testis
IV	abundant coarse, curly hair; breast, areola, papilla → 2° mound	adult config. of hair; ↑ size of glans penis; darker scrotum
V	ADULT →	

Kawasaki Disease (mucocutaneous lymph node syndrome)

- unknown origin; kids < 5 y.o.
- abrupt onset of high fever; arthritis, conjunctivitis, fissured lips, erythematous rash, painful peripheral edema,
- may develop coronary arteritis → possibly aneurysms & MI

Advanced Life Support for the USMLE Step 2, by Flynn et al.
Lippincott–Raven Publishers © 1997.

CHAPTER 5

Obstetrics and Gynecology

Ben Yeh

Study Hints

- Obstetrics is heavily tested.
- The differential diagnosis of abnormal vaginal bleeding is very high yield.
- For gynecologic neoplasms, the classic presentations, epidemiology, and patterns of spread are high yield. Staging systems and chemotherapy regimens are low yield.
- The anatomy of the pelvis and perineum is low yield.
- Hormone changes during the menstrual cycle are low yield.
- Unusual types of multiple gestations are low yield.

Obstetrics

TERMINOLOGY

- A **premature delivery** is delivery between 20 and 37 weeks of an infant weighing 500 to 2500 g.
- An abortion is delivery before 20 weeks.
- **G#P#** is the annotation the USMLE Step 2 uses to describe obstetric history.

  - **G** means gravidity, the total number of pregnancies that the patient has had.
  - **P** means parity, the number of pregnancies carried at least 20 weeks.
- Neither G nor P is affected by the number of fetuses carried during any pregnancy. For example, a nonpregnant woman who has had one abortion and carried triplets to term is a G2P1.

GENERAL OBSTETRICS POINTS

- The #1 cause of maternal death in the U.S. remains **pulmonary embolism.** It is usually associated with deep venous thrombosis. **Treat high risk patients with heparin, not warfarin.** Warfarin is a teratogen.
- IgG is the only immunoglobulin that crosses the placenta.
- IgA is the only immunoglobulin in bre**A**st milk and colostrum.
- The two **positive signs of pregnancy** are detection of a fetal heart beat and recognition of fetal movements. They are considered the only 100% reliable indicators of pregnancy.
- A cyanotic-looking bluish cervix and vaginal wall is **Chadwick's sign,** one of the presumptive signs of pregnancy.

PHYSIOLOGIC CHANGES OF PREGNANCY

- The physiologic changes of pregnancy are depicted in Figure 5-1.

ECTOPIC PREGNANCY

- The incidence of ectopic pregnancy has risen.
- **95% of ectopic pregnancies occur in the fallopian tube.** Most sources say that the **ampulla** is the most common site.
- Risk factors for ectopic pregnancy include **a history of pelvic inflammatory disease (salpingitis),** prior ectopic pregnancy, tubal ligation, and use of IUDs.

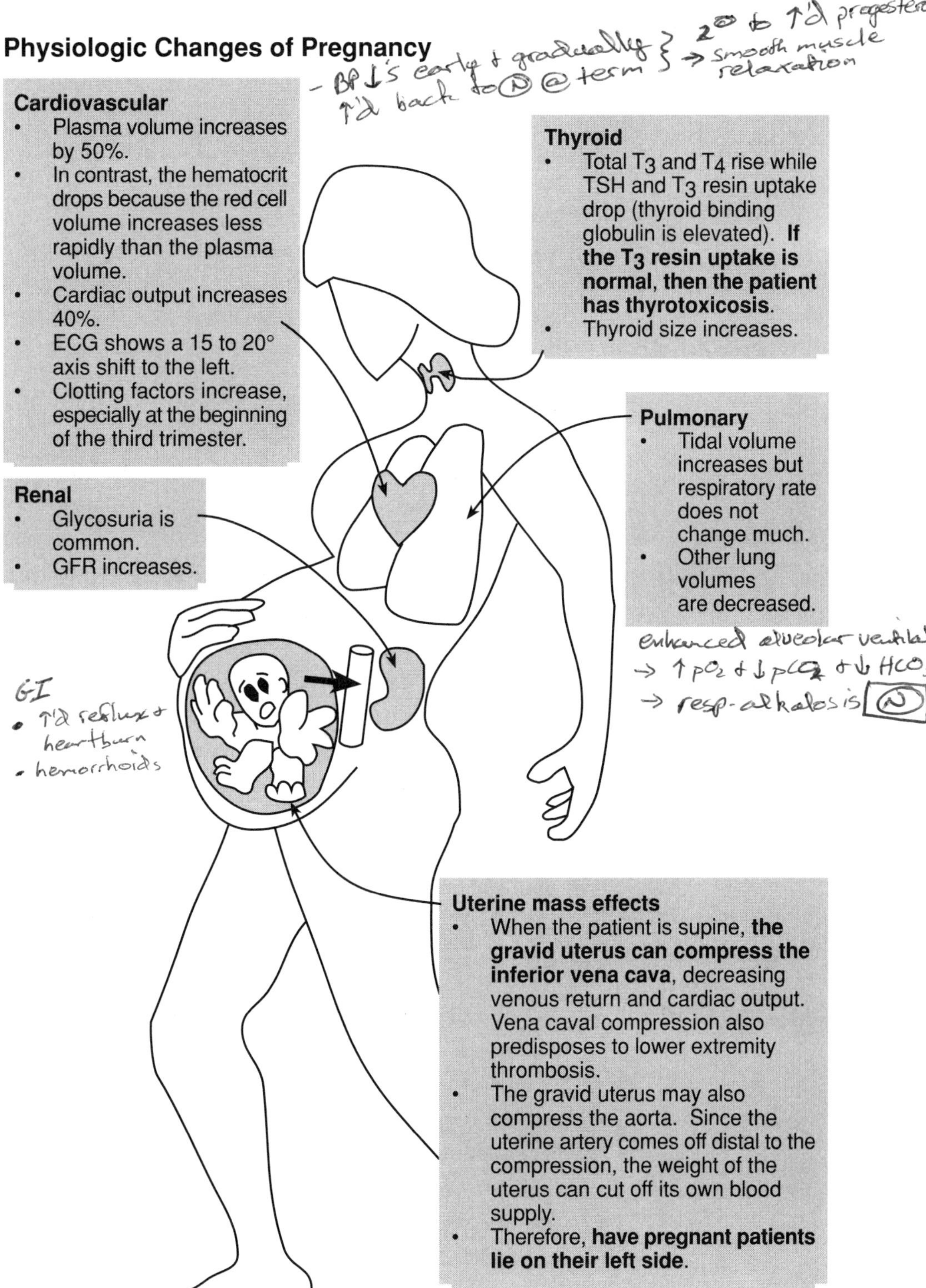
Physiologic Changes of Pregnancy
Cardiovascular
• Plasma volume increases by 50%.
• In contrast, the hematocrit drops because the red cell volume increases less rapidly than the plasma volume.
• Cardiac output increases 40%.
• ECG shows a 15 to 20° axis shift to the left.
• Clotting factors increase, especially at the beginning of the third trimester.
Thyroid
• Total T_3 and T_4 rise while TSH and T_3 resin uptake drop (thyroid binding globulin is elevated). **If the T_3 resin uptake is normal, then the patient has thyrotoxicosis**.
• Thyroid size increases.
Pulmonary
• Tidal volume increases but respiratory rate does not change much.
• Other lung volumes are decreased.
Renal
• Glycosuria is common.
• GFR increases.
Uterine mass effects
• When the patient is supine, **the gravid uterus can compress the inferior vena cava**, decreasing venous return and cardiac output. Vena caval compression also predisposes to lower extremity thrombosis.
• The gravid uterus may also compress the aorta. Since the uterine artery comes off distal to the compression, the weight of the uterus can cut off its own blood supply.
• Therefore, **have pregnant patients lie on their left side**.

Figure 5-1

- The classic symptom triad is amenorrhea, abnormal vaginal bleeding, and abdominal pain.
- **An elevated β-hCG in the absence of uterine pregnancy by ultrasound** is usually considered diagnostic.
- Mothers can bleed to death if their ectopic pregnancy ruptures.

SPONTANEOUS ABORTION

- Spontaneous abortion occurs in about 10% to 15% of recognized pregnancies and about 50% of all conceptions.
- Risk factors for spontaneous abortion include prior spontaneous abortions, infection, exposure to teratogens, smoking, alcohol use, and lupus.
- **Threatened abortion** is a pregnancy complicated by vaginal bleeding prior to the 20th week.
- **Inevitable abortion** is a pregnancy complicated by both vaginal bleeding and lower abdominal cramps. The cervix is often partially dilated.
- **Incomplete abortion** is an inevitable abortion with passage of part of the conceptus.
- **Complete abortion** involves passage of all products of conception.
- **Missed abortion** is a fetus that has died but remains in the uterus for a few weeks. The mother is at risk for DIC.

PRENATAL CARE

- **The first ultrasound is the most accurate** for determining fetal age. First ultrasounds are usually performed at 16 to 20 weeks.
- The top causes of an elevated alpha-fetoprotein are **multiple gestation** and **open neural tube defects** such as anencephaly or spina bifida.
- After 20 weeks, the fundal height in centimeters should be roughly equivalent to the gestational age in weeks. Fundal height is measured from the symphysis pubis to the top of the fundus.
- Intrauterine growth retardation (IUGR) is a fetal size that is small for gestational age. One of the earliest ultrasound

indicators of IUGR is a **fetal abdominal circumference** below the 10th percentile.

PREECLAMPSIA AND ECLAMPSIA

- Risk factors include young age, first pregnancy, and large uterus (large babies, multiple gestation, polyhydramnios, and molar pregnancy).
- The **preeclampsia triad** is proteinuria, hypertension, and edema of the hands and face. Severe preeclampsia is marked by **proteinuria >5 g/day,** BP >160/110, or systemic symptoms.
- **Eclampsia is preeclampsia with grand mal seizures.** The seizures may occur before, during, or *after* delivery. Half occur during labor.
- Preeclamptics and eclamptics are at risk for the HELLP syndrome, which includes **h**emolytic anemia, **e**levated **l**iver enzymes, and a **l**ow **p**latelet count.
- Treat all cases with bed rest.
- Treat hypertension with **hydralazine or β-blockers.**
- Treat seizures with **magnesium sulfate.**
- The definitive treatment of preeclampsia is **delivery.**

DIABETES IN PREGNANCY

- All pregnant women are screened for gestational diabetes with a glucose tolerance test.
- Tight control of blood glucose is mandatory even before conception in known diabetics. Tight control lowers the risk for most maternal and fetal complications.
- Maternal complications of diabetes include polyhydramnios and preeclampsia.
- Fetal complications of diabetes include **macrosomia** (big baby) and congenital anomalies.

MULTIPLE GESTATION

- Multiple gestation results in a **50% premature birth rate.** Mothers are at higher risk for complications such as hypertensive disease and hemorrhage.

SUBSTANCE ABUSE

- Cocaine abuse increases the risk of hypertension, placental abruption, and fetal demise. **Stop cocaine use during pregnancy.**
- Heroin abuse, on the other hand, may cause fetal morbidity upon stopping the drug due to fetal narcotic withdrawal. **Maintain the patient on methadone** during pregnancy.

TERATOGENS

Teratogen	*Notes*
Isotretinoin	Contraceptives and repeated **β-hCG pregnancy tests** required for fertile female patients starting isotretinoin for acne
Thalidomide	Limb defects
Diethylstilbestrol	Clear cell adenocarcinoma of the vagina
Ethanol	Fetal alcohol syndrome consisting of mental retardation; growth deficiency; cardiac defects; and **craniofacial defects** including microcephaly, short palpebral fissures, micrognathia, and poorly formed ears

MISCELLANEOUS ILLNESSES OF PREGNANCY

- **Iron deficiency anemia** accounts for 80% of anemia during pregnancy.
- Hyperemesis gravidarum occurs in the first trimester. It is generally self-limiting. Treat with reassurance and multiple small feedings. IV fluids and antiemetics may be required.

PLACENTAL AND UTERINE ANOMALIES

- Figure 5-2 illustrates some placental and uterine anomalies.

Placental and Uterine Abnormalities

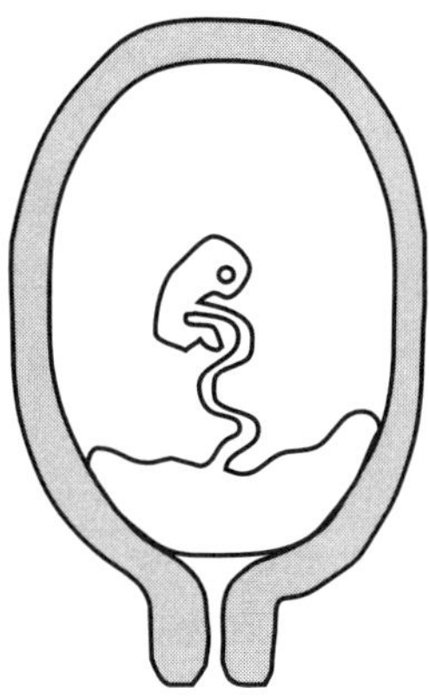

Placenta previa

- Risk factors include prior cesarean sections and multiparity.
- **Painless vaginal bleeding is the hallmark**.
- **Do not do a pelvic exam on patients with significant third trimester bleeding** until you first rule out placenta previa by transabdominal ultrasound. Otherwise you may precipitate massive hemorrhage.
- **Bedrest** with or without hospitalization is mandatory.
- The patient should not engage in sexual intercourse (this is called 'pelvic rest'). The patient may also be advised to avoid nipple stimulation, as oxytocin release secondary to nipple stimulation can cause uterine contractions.
- Uterine contractions should be controlled with magnesium sulfate, not β-blockers.
- Ultimately, **delivery by cesarean section** is mandatory.

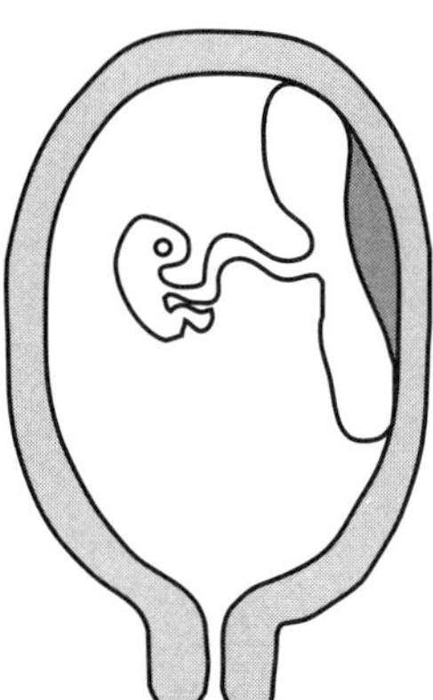

Placental abruption

- Placental abruption is premature separation of the normally implanted placenta.
- Risk factors include **hypertension** (including preeclampsia), previous abruption, trauma, rapid decompression of the uterus (polyhydramnios, delivery of one twin), and tobacco or cocaine use.
- Placental abruption is associated with **painful vaginal bleeding**, back pain, and a tetanic contracted 'board-like' uterus. Abruptions will not cause vaginal bleeding if they do not communicate with the cervical os.
- Abruptions are an obstetric emergency. The mother and fetus may rapidly die of hemorrhage, and further contractions may worsen the abruption. Some sources advise cesarean section even for small abruptions.

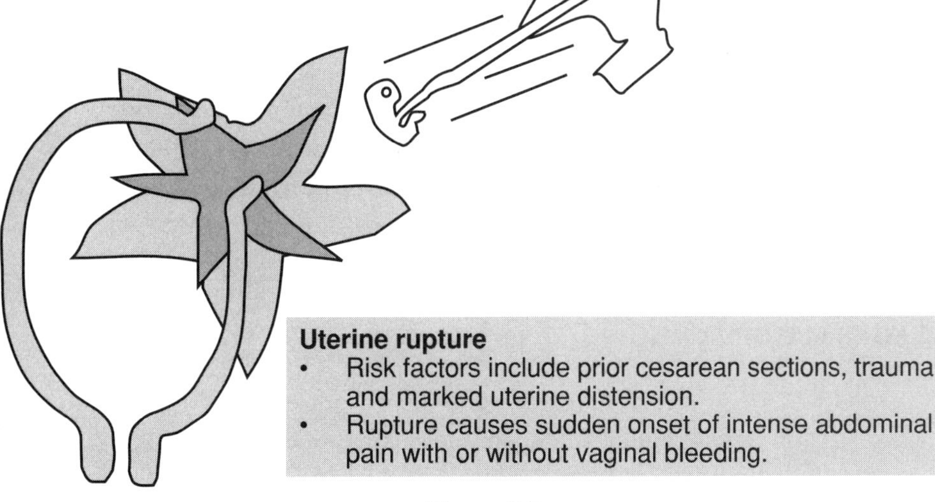

Uterine rupture

- Risk factors include prior cesarean sections, trauma, and marked uterine distension.
- Rupture causes sudden onset of intense abdominal pain with or without vaginal bleeding.

Figure 5-2

FETAL WELL-BEING

- There are four basic tests of fetal well-being. These tests are presented below in the order that they would normally be done.

1. **Maternal assessment of fetal movement** suggests fetal well-being if the mother feels at least ten fetal movements in 12 hours.
2. The **nonstress test** (NST) determines if the fetal heart accelerates when the fetus moves. A healthy fetus will have at least two significant accelerations in a 20-minute interval. A significant acceleration is an increase in heart rate of at least 15 beats per minute for 15 seconds or more. **Normal NSTs are called reactive.**
3. **Ultrasonography** evaluates amniotic fluid volume, fetal breathing, and fetal movement. A **biophysical profile** is a nonstress test combined with ultrasonography.
4. The **contraction stress test** uses oxytocin infusion or nipple stimulation to induce mild uterine contractions. It is done when the nonstress test is nonreactive (abnormal). If late decelerations are observed, the test is called positive and the baby should be delivered.

AMNIOTIC FLUID

- Amniotic fluid is in a state of dynamic balance. It is primarily fetal urine **generated by fetal kidneys.** It is **removed by fetal swallowing** and by absorption into the maternal circulation.
- Oligohydramnios is a marked deficiency of amniotic fluid. Oligohydramnios suggests **intrauterine growth retardation** (60% of the time), fetal stress, or renal agenesis.
- Polyhydramnios is excessive amniotic fluid. It results in an enlarged uterus. Polyhydramnios is associated with **duodenal atresia, CNS anomalies, hydrops fetalis,** maternal diabetes, and tracheoesophageal fistula.

FETAL LUNG MATURITY

- Fetal lungs are considered mature when the ratio of lecithin to sphingomyelin in amniotic fluid is >2:1.

- Corticosteroids stimulate the production of surfactant and the maturation of alveolar type II cells. Corticosteroids are often given to pregnant mothers when delivery is required but the fetal lungs are not yet mature.

PREMATURE RUPTURE OF MEMBRANES

- Rupture of membranes is premature when it occurs before the onset of labor.
- Premature rupture of membranes (PROM) is diagnosed by history and sterile speculum examination. **Ferning** of vaginal fluid is virtually diagnostic. Other signs of PROM include vaginal pooling and a positive nitrazine test.
- **Fetal lung maturity is a key issue in PROM.** If the fetus is ≥36 weeks, wait a few hours before inducing labor. If the fetus is ≦35 weeks, wait 16 hours before inducing labor to promote lung maturation, and give the infant surfactant at birth.
- Prophylactic antibiotics should be given if the fetus is <37 weeks.
- If mom becomes febrile or septic after PROM, assume chorioamnionitis is present. Treat with ampicillin, gentamicin, *and* clindamycin or metronidazole. If triple therapy is not an option, choose ampicillin only. Do not give tocolytics.

LABOR

- **True labor** is defined as regular uterine contractions occurring at least every 5 minutes, with each contraction lasting at least 30 seconds.
- **Braxton Hicks contractions,** or false labor, are uterine contractions in the third trimester that do not meet the criteria for true labor.
- Treat premature labor with **pelvic rest** and **hydration.** If labor continues, tocolyze with **magnesium, ritodrine, or terbutaline.** Ritodrine and terbutaline are β_2-agonists.

BREECH PRESENTATION

- Different types of breech presentation are shown in Figure 5-3.

Breech Presentation

- Uterine anomalies and prematurity are the major risk factors for breech presentation.
- External version may be attempted after 37 weeks. Internal version is no longer attempted due to risk of uterine rupture.
- Breech presentations are usually delivered by cesarean section due to high risk of umbilical cord prolapse, birth asphyxia, and dystocia.
- **Frank breech** (butt first with both feet straight up) is the only breech presentation which may be delivered vaginally.

May deliver vaginally

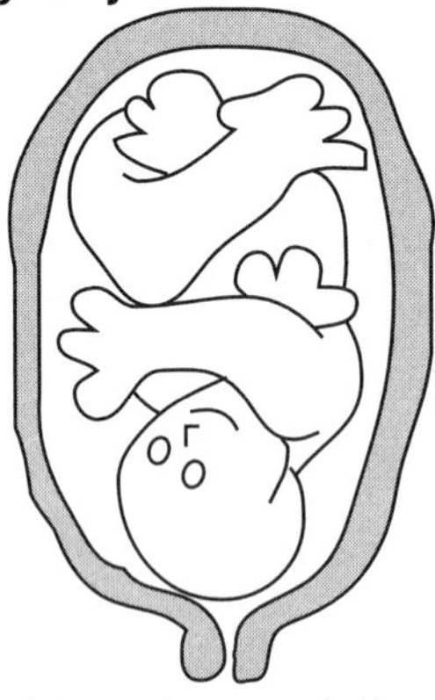

Normal presentation

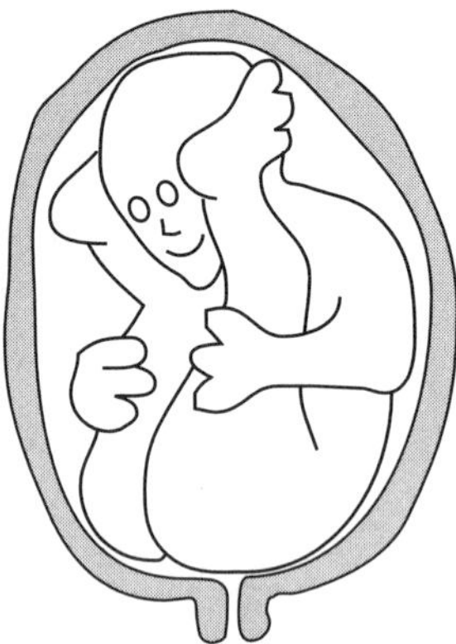

Frank breech

Deliver by cesarean section

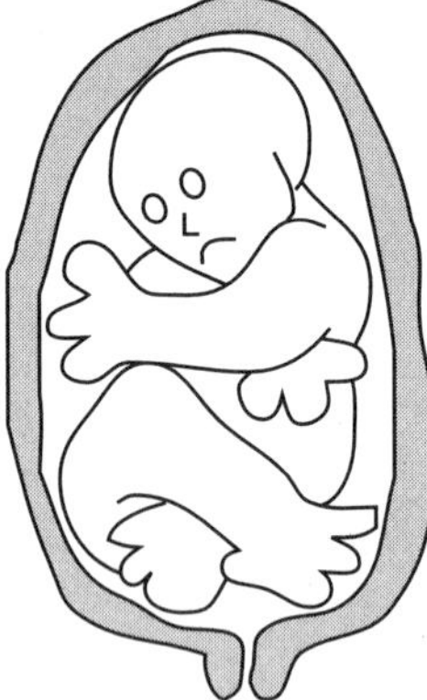

Complete breech

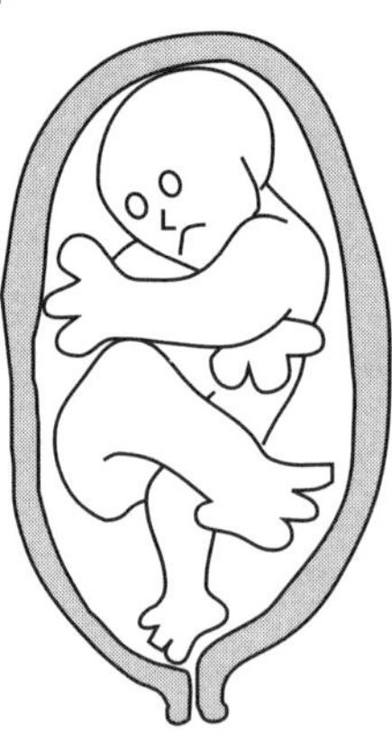

Footling breech

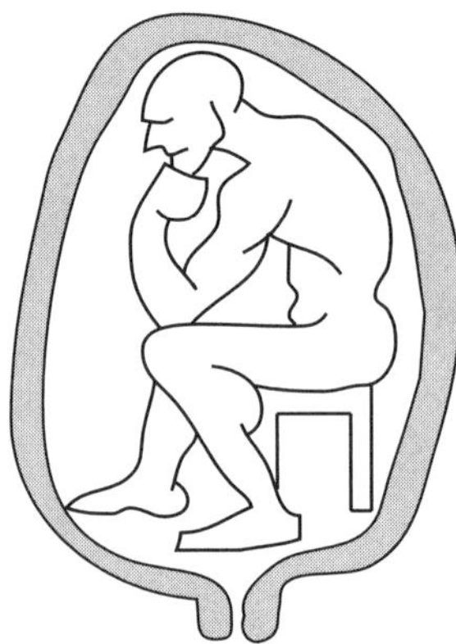

Double footling breech

Figure 5-3

THE STAGES OF LABOR

Stage	*Duration (1st baby)*	*Description*
First	6–18 h	Onset of true labor through cervical effacement to full cervical dilation
Second	30 min to 3 h	From complete cervical dilation to birth of the baby
Third	0–30 min	From birth of the baby to delivery of the placenta
Fourth	About 6 h	From placental delivery to stabilization of the mother

- **Station** is the distance of the presenting part above or below the level of the ischial spines. Zero station is at the level of the ischial spines. 3+ station is 3 cm *below* the ischial spines.
- **Forceps or suction delivery** is the first-line intervention when fetal distress is noted and the fetus is 2+ station or lower (3+, 4+, etc.).
- **Arrest** may occur during the active phase of labor. Arrest is 2 hours without progression of cervical dilatation. **Cephalopelvic disproportion** and fetal malpresentation must be ruled out by exam. If the exam is normal, give oxytocin to correct uterine hypotony.

FETAL MONITORING DURING LABOR

- There are three main types of decelerations seen on fetal heart rate and uterine contraction strips (FHR-UC strips). These decelerations are classified according to their relation to uterine contractions.
- **Early decelerations** suggest **head compression** during uterine contraction. They are not associated with fetal distress.

- **Variable decelerations** suggest **umbilical cord compression. Lie mom on her left side and give her oxygen.** If the fetal scalp pH drops, rapid delivery is required.
- **Late decelerations** suggest uteroplacental insufficiency such as may occur with hypotension, abruption, or rupture of the uterus. Give oxygen and tocolytics, and **deliver the baby as soon as possible.**
- You are not asked to read actual FHR-UC strips.

STDs, INFECTION, AND LABOR

- **Active herpes requires a cesarean section.** For USMLE Step 2 purposes, **all other STDs may be delivered vaginally.**
- Mothers infected with HIV should receive **zidovudine (AZT)** in the last two trimesters and during delivery. AZT reduces transmission to the fetus. The newborn should also be treated with AZT for the first 6 weeks of life.
- If mom has positive hepatitis B antigen titers, the infant should receive the hepatitis B vaccine and hepatitis B hyperimmune globulin at birth.
- Patients with syphilis, gonorrhea, or chlamydia should receive antibiotics as soon as they are diagnosed. Treat chlamydia in pregnant women with **erythromycin,** not doxycycline. Make sure the infant receives eye prophylaxis with erythromycin or silver nitrate.
- Vaginal Group B *Streptococcus* carriage is very common. Most protocols do not call for ampicillin during labor. Symptomatic babies are given ampicillin after birth.
- Rarely, condyloma acuminata (venereal warts) may be so extensive that cesarean section is preferable.

POSTPARTUM HEMORRHAGE

- **The great majority of postpartum hemorrhages are due to uterine atony.** Treat with dilute oxytocin infusion. If oxytocin fails, use ergonovine.
- The second most common cause of postpartum hemorrhage is genital tract trauma.

- If the mother continues to bleed several hours postpartum, then regardless of the consistency of the uterus she most likely has **retained products of conception.** The uterine cavity must be explored or imaged by ultrasound.
- If the mother continues to bleed 2 to 3 days postpartum, then she most likely has **puerperal endometritis or sepsis.** Explore the cervical os. If there are any signs of infection or sepsis, treat with antibiotics.

Gynecology

VAGINOSES

- **Bacterial vaginosis** is marked by a heavy gray malodorous vaginal discharge. *Gardnerella* is considered the most common cause. Wet mounts reveal **clue cells,** which are squamous cells with chewed-up edges. Treat the patient and any sexual partners with **metronidazole.**
- ***Candida albicans*** infections are marked by itching and a cottage cheese-like white discharge. Pseudohyphae and spores are seen on KOH prep. Treat with **nystatin,** miconazole, clotrimazole, or terconazole.

SEXUALLY TRANSMITTED DISEASES

- Trichomonas is marked by a yellow-green vaginal discharge. Wet mounts reveal **motile trichomonads.** A "strawberry cervix" (petechiae on the cervix) may be seen. Treat the patient and her partners with **metronidazole.**
- Condyloma acuminata, or venereal warts, are asymptomatic cauliflower-like lesions caused by human papilloma virus types 6 and 11. A young girl with multiple warty growths on her vulva which look like bunches of grapes has **sarcoma botryoides,** not condyloma.
- Herpes genitalis presents as painful vesicles on the perineum and external genitalia. Herpes simplex type 2 is the most common cause. **Acyclovir during the initial attack** shortens the duration of both symptoms and viral shedding.

- Gonorrhea is often asymptomatic in women but may present with dysuria, urinary frequency, or a purulent urethral discharge. Males generally have worse symptoms with creamy blood-tinged urethral discharges. Gram stain and culture demonstrate **gram-negative diplococci within polymorphonuclear leukocytes.** Treat with **IM ceftriaxone** *and* **oral doxycycline.** The ceftriaxone is for the gonorrhea; the doxycycline is for the presumed *Chlamydia* co-infection seen in up to half of these patients.
- Chlamydia is often asymptomatic but may cause symptomatic cervicitis or pelvic inflammatory disease (salpingitis). The diagnosis is usually presumptive. Treat with **doxycycline.** *Chlamydia* species also cause lymphogranuloma venereum.
- The incidence of syphilis is on the rise. Transmission to the fetus can occur at any stage. Treat with **penicillin.**

STAGES OF SYPHILIS

Stage of Syphilis	*Time*	*Symptoms and Signs*
Primary	2–6 wk	Firm **painless ulcer** on the genitalia
Secondary	1–6 mo	**Positive serologic test for syphilis** Generalized maculopapular skin rash Mucous membrane lesions (condyloma lata) Fever, meningitis, and arthritis
Tertiary	Years	**Aortic aneurysms and aortic regurgitation** Tumors (gummas) of the skin, bones, and liver CNS disorders

INFERTILITY

- Figure 5-4 illustrates some causes of infertility.

Infertility

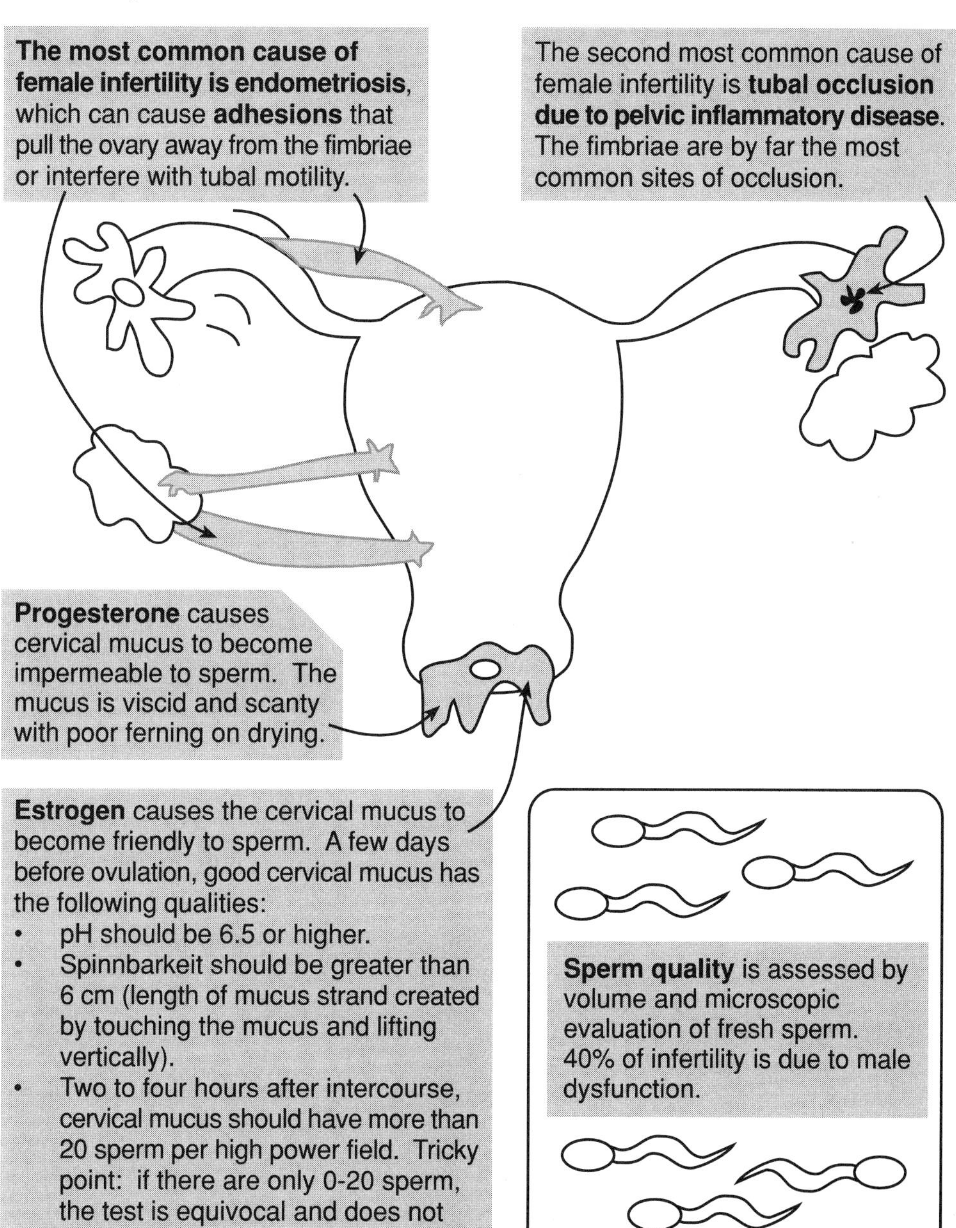

The most common cause of female infertility is endometriosis, which can cause **adhesions** that pull the ovary away from the fimbriae or interfere with tubal motility.
The second most common cause of female infertility is **tubal occlusion due to pelvic inflammatory disease**. The fimbriae are by far the most common sites of occlusion.
Progesterone causes cervical mucus to become impermeable to sperm. The mucus is viscid and scanty with poor ferning on drying.
Estrogen causes the cervical mucus to become friendly to sperm. A few days before ovulation, good cervical mucus has the following qualities:
• pH should be 6.5 or higher.
• Spinnbarkeit should be greater than 6 cm (length of mucus strand created by touching the mucus and lifting vertically).
• Two to four hours after intercourse, cervical mucus should have more than 20 sperm per high power field. Tricky point: if there are only 0-20 sperm, the test is equivocal and does not imply that the sperm quality is bad.
Sperm quality is assessed by volume and microscopic evaluation of fresh sperm. 40% of infertility is due to male dysfunction.

Figure 5-4

Gynecologic Neoplasms

- Believe it or not, these are heavily tested.

ENDOMETRIOSIS

- Look for questions on endometriosis.
- Endometriosis refers to endometrial glands and stroma existing outside of the uterine cavity. The ovaries are the most common sites.
- The main risk factor is nulliparity.
- The classic triad of endometriosis is dysmenorrhea, dyspareunia, and dyschezia (difficulty defecating) that cycles with menses. Pre- and postmenstrual **spotting** are common.
- **Tender adnexal masses and tender nodules on the uterosacral ligaments are classic.**
- Laparoscopy typically reveals **chocolate-colored cysts** on the ovary and brown or blue spots on the peritoneal surfaces. Fibrosis and scarring can occur.
- **Oral contraceptives** with progesterone are given for mild disease.
- Infertility due to endometriosis is treated with excision and lysis of adhesions. Fertility is restored in about half of patients.
- Endometriosis usually regresses after menopause.

ENDOMETRIAL CANCER

- The major risk factor for endometrial cancer is estrogen unopposed by progesterone. Such a state occurs with obesity, nulliparity, late menopause, some postmenopausal estrogen therapies, and estrogen-only birth control pills.
- Median age of onset is 60 years.
- The major symptom is abnormal vaginal bleeding, especially **postmenopausal bleeding.**
- **Spread is by direct local extension.** Once through the uterine serosa, endometrial cancer spreads to the local pelvic lymph nodes and then to the periaortic lymph nodes.
- Treat surgically.

CERVICAL CANCER

- **The incidence of invasive cervical cancer has decreased dramatically** since the 1930s, mainly due to the wide use of the **Papanicolaou smear.** Pap smears allow for early detection and subsequent cure.
- Risk factors include early sexual intercourse, multiple sexual partners, high parity, young age of first pregnancy or marriage, and low socioeconomic status.
- **Human papilloma virus** is associated with cervical neoplasia.
- Pap smears should be done annually starting at first coitus or age 18. Patients with no risk factors who have had two normal Pap smears may be screened every 2 to 5 years.
- **False negative Pap smears are common.** If a woman has a positive Pap smear, she should be evaluated regardless of the results of subsequent smears.
- Treat carcinoma in situ (cervical intraepithelial neoplasia, or CIN) with cervical conization, hysterectomy, cryotherapy, CO_2 laser, or electrocoagulation.
- Cervical cancer spreads by **direct local extension** and by lymphatics to the **periaortic lymph nodes.**
- Advanced disease is treated with surgery or radiation. Chemotherapy outcomes are poor.
- **Invasive cancer in pregnancy detected prior to 22 weeks requires abortion** and surgery or radiation. All other stages, including carcinoma in situ and frankly invasive cancer detected after 22 weeks, can wait until after delivery.

OVARIAN CANCER

- **Ovarian cancer is the number one cause of *gynecologic* cancer death.** It is the fifth most common cancer in U.S. females.
- Peak incidence is in the 40s and 50s. Ovarian cancer is usually advanced at the time of diagnosis.
- Risk factors include **nulliparity** and a family history of ovarian *or* endometrial cancer.
- Signs and symptoms include **ascites,** abdominal discomfort, and atypical vaginal bleeding. Watch for the woman with ascites and a cancer profile.

- **Spread is by peritoneal seeding.**
- Treat with surgical debulking followed by chemotherapy.

FOLLICULAR CYSTS

- **Follicular cysts** occur with menses. They are benign, but they must be distinguished from ovarian cancer.
- They can be **up to 8 cm** in diameter.
- They are usually asymptomatic.
- If a simple cyst is found on the ovary, follow it for one menstrual period. It should regress.

VULVAR CANCER

- **Squamous cell carcinoma** is the most common type of cancer of the vulva and vagina.
- Postmenopausal women are most commonly affected.
- Spread is mainly by direct local extension. However, lymph node metastases do occur in a progressive fashion going from the inguinal nodes to the femoral nodes and then the pelvic nodes.
- **Wide excision** is the mainstay of treatment for *vulvar* cancer.
- Radiotherapy is the preferred treatment for the rare vaginal cancer.
- Melanoma is the #2 cancer of the vulva. Prognosis is poor.

GESTATIONAL TROPHOBLASTIC NEOPLASIA

- The benign form is called a hydatidiform mole. The malignant form is called choriocarcinoma. All forms may embolize to the lung or other tissues.
- A hydatidiform mole looks like a **bunch of grapes.** Signs and symptoms include a **large uterus for dates, abnormally high β-hCG levels, and passage of grape-like vesicles** out of the vagina. Keep in mind that multiple gestation may also present with high β-hCG levels and a large uterus for dates.
- A **"snowstorm" appearance** of the mole on ultrasonography is pathognomonic.
- Treat by evacuating the uterus. Then **follow the β-hCG titers.** If they continue to rise, give **methotrexate.**

LEIOMYOMA (UTERINE FIBROID)

- **Leiomyomas are the most common uterine tumor.** They are benign tumors of smooth muscle.
- **Pedunculated submucosal leiomyomas may protrude into the uterine cavity and even out of the cervix.**
- Although benign, leiomyomas can cause problems by obstruction or mass effect. They may also ulcerate into the mucosa and cause abnormal uterine bleeding (metrorrhagia) or excessive bleeding during periods (menorrhagia).
- Leiomyomas are estrogen dependent and may grow rapidly during pregnancy.

MENOPAUSE

- The mean age of menopause is 51 years.
- Menopause occurs when all ova become atretic. The ovary then no longer responds well to gonadotropins. Gonadotropin levels increase as estrogen and progesterone levels fall.
- Perimenopausal symptoms include anovulation, menstrual irregularity, emotional changes, and hot flashes.
- Atrophic vaginitis, osteoporosis, and atherosclerosis are more common after menopause.
- The most common causes of postmenopausal bleeding are exogenous estrogens and atrophic endometritis or vaginitis. Endometrial cancer and other neoplasms are the next most common causes.

Dysmenorrhea

1° Dysmenorrhea - ideopathic or ∅ identifiable GYN cause
xs production of prostaglandin $F_2\alpha$

2° - organic basis

Abnormal Uterine Bleeding

1) amenorrhea – lack of menses
2) menorrhagia - reg. intervals but > 7days duration
3) metorrhagia - freq. + irregular
4) menometorrhagia - irreg. + > 7d.
5) polymenorrhea - reg. but @ intervals < 21d
6) intermenstrual -

Anatomic causes

- leiomyomata
- infection
- cervical + endometrial polyps
- neoplasia

Amenorrhea

1° - lack of menses by age 14 + s̄ 2° sex characteristics
or by age 16 + c̄ " "

2° - absence of menses for 3cycles or 6mo

look for uterine or outflow disorders, ovarian disorders, pituitary disorders, + CNS disorders

Advanced Life Support for the USMLE Step 2, by Flynn et al.
Lippincott–Raven Publishers © 1997.

CHAPTER 6

Internal Medicine

Matt Flynn

Study Hints

- Do not study internal medicine heavily unless you are strong in the other disciplines.
- Outpatient medicine is high yield relative to inpatient medicine.
- Several questions will present a list of tests that are normally ordered as a group, then ask which test should be ordered *first.* Select the test that will confirm or disprove the most likely diagnosis.
- You will be presented with a great deal of lab data. Blood counts, liver function tests, and urinalyses are particularly popular.
- Race is never included in descriptions.
- Many clinical vignettes give height and weight. Skip them unless the weight is over 200 pounds (90 kg) or under 100 pounds (45 kg).

Vitamin Deficiencies

- Vitamin deficiencies are very popular. *All* of the following are fair game, even vitamin E.

VITAMIN B_{12} IN DETAIL

- Vitamin B_{12} and folate deficiency both cause **megaloblastic, macrocytic anemia** (MCV >100) with **hypersegmented neutrophils.**
- B_{12} deficiency also causes **peripheral neuropathy, dementia,** posterior column damage leading to position and vibration sense problems, and occasionally pancytopenia.
- **Pernicious anemia is the #1 cause of B_{12} deficiency.** Atrophic gastritis is a hallmark of pernicious anemia.
- Other causes of B_{12} deficiency include stomach or ileal resection, overgrowth of bacteria in a blind loop of bowel or a Meckel's diverticulum, strict vegetarianism, and the fish tapeworm *Diphyllobothrium latum* (no kidding).
- A **low serum B_{12} level** is diagnostic.
- The treatment is intramuscular B_{12}.
- Vitamin B_{12} is found in meats, fish, and dairy products.

FOLATE

- Like B_{12} deficiency, folate deficiency causes **megaloblastic anemia** and **hypersegmented neutrophils.** However, it does not cause neurologic manifestations.
- **Do not give folate until B_{12} deficiency is ruled out.**
- **Dietary insufficiency is the #1 cause of folate deficiency.** Alcoholics and pregnant women are particularly vulnerable.
- Citrus fruits and green leafy vegetables contain lots of folate.

OTHER WATER-SOLUBLE VITAMINS

- **Alcoholics** get these deficiencies.
- Isoniazid causes B_6 deficiency.
- Poor diet is a major cause of vitamin C deficiency.

Vitamin	*Signs of Deficiency and Notes*
Thiamine (B_1)	Wet beri-beri involves high output heart failure. Dry beri-beri involves symmetric neuropathy with pain.

	Wernicke's encephalopathy involves the triad of ataxia, confusion, and ophthalmoplegia.
	Korsakoff's syndrome involves anterograde amnesia.
	For Board purposes, **always give thiamine to alcoholics before IV dextrose or glucose.**
Niacin (B_3)	The **3 Ds of pellagra** are **d**iarrhea, **d**ementia, and **d**ermatitis.
Pyridoxine (B_6)	Pyridoxine deficiency presents with peripheral neuropathy, microcytic anemia, and sometimes seizures.
C (Ascorbic acid)	Signs of scurvy include bleeding gums, perifollicular petechiae, anemia, and impaired wound healing. Patients' bones ache due to periosteal hemorrhage.

FAT-SOLUBLE VITAMINS

- **Malabsorption** causes fat-soluble vitamin deficiencies.
- Warfarin is the #1 cause of vitamin K deficiency.

Vitamin	*Signs of Deficiency and Notes*
A	Night blindness and scaly rash
D	Rickets (kids): defective bone growth and leg bowing Osteomalacia (adults): osteopenia and bone tenderness
E	Ataxia, areflexia and ophthalmoplegia
K	Prolonged prothrombin time, petechiae and hemorrhage

Autosomal Dominant Diseases

FAMILIAL HYPERCHOLESTEROLEMIA

- Familial hypercholesterolemia is caused by **absent or defective LDL receptors.**

- LDL cholesterol will be very high, often >300 mg/dL.
- Patients have xanthomas and develop severe atherosclerosis at a young age.

MARFAN'S SYNDROME

- Marfan's syndrome is due to defective connective tissue.
- Patients are tailor-made for professional basketball—they are tall with long limbs and hyperextensible joints.
- **Aortic aneurysm** and **aortic dissection** are dreaded complications.
- Aortic valve insufficiency and mitral valve prolapse are common.

HUNTINGTON'S DISEASE

- Huntington's disease causes progressive dementia and choreiform movements. Onset is in the 30s or 40s.

NEUROFIBROMATOSIS TYPES I AND II

- Neurofibromatosis type I (von Recklinghausen's disease) is characterized by café-au-lait spots and neurofibromas. The neurofibromas are mostly on the skin, but **acoustic neuromas** can occur.
- The hallmark of neurofibromatosis type II is bilateral acoustic neuromas.

HEREDITARY SPHEROCYTOSIS

- Hereditary spherocytosis predisposes to intermittent hemolytic anemia.
- Defective red blood cells are destroyed in the spleen.
- **Splenectomy** cures the anemia.

VON WILLEBRAND'S DISEASE

- Von Willebrand's disease is the **most common hereditary bleeding disorder.**

- Von Willebrand's factor carries factor VIII and mediates platelet adhesion.
- **Bleeding time** and PTT are prolonged. PT is normal.
- In contrast, in the X-linked disease hemophilia A (factor VIII deficiency), the PTT is prolonged but bleeding time is normal.

Vasculitides

- Look for questions on vasculitides.

WEGENER'S GRANULOMATOSIS

- The classic triad of Wegener's granulomatosis is **sinusitis, pneumonitis, and glomerulonephritis.** Patients typically present with recurrent sinus infections, shortness of breath, cough, and hemoptysis.
- **The lungs are involved.**
- Middle-aged males are most commonly affected.
- Treat with prednisone and cyclophosphamide.

POLYARTERITIS NODOSA

- **Lung involvement is rare.** PAN can cause vascular lesions in almost any other organ.
- Kidney failure is common.
- Middle-aged males are most commonly affected.
- Onset can be abrupt. Patients undergo exacerbations and remissions. Exacerbations involve fever, weight loss, and weakness.
- Treat with steroids.

TAKAYASU'S ARTERITIS

- Takayasu's arteritis causes vascular insufficiency in the upper extremities and in the carotid distribution.

- **Numb or cold arms** may be present, especially if the radial pulse is absent. Takayasu's arteritis is also called **pulseless disease.**
- Young women are most commonly affected.

THROMBOANGIITIS OBLITERANS

- Thromboangiitis obliterans leads to **claudication** in all limbs.
- **Raynaud's phenomenon** is a frequent finding.
- Middle-aged **male smokers** get the disease.

Headache

MIGRAINE

- Migraines usually present as a **unilateral throbbing headache** preceded by photophobia, nausea, or flashes of light.
- The disease first appears in adolescence or young adulthood and can be familial.
- Treat with **sumatriptan,** caffeine, and ergotamines.
- Use **propranolol** or amitriptyline for prophylaxis.

CLUSTER HEADACHE

- Typically, severe **unilateral orbital pain** awakens the patient from sleep. Eye irritation and Horner's syndrome are sometimes present.
- Cluster headaches occur most commonly in **middle-aged males.** They appear daily in clusters lasting weeks.
- Treat with **100% oxygen** with or without ergotamines.

TEMPORAL ARTERITIS

- Temporal arteritis (giant cell arteritis) typically presents in elderly patients as a **unilateral throbbing headache** with temporal artery tenderness.
- Fever, anemia, and an **elevated ESR** are common findings.

- Half of patients also have **polymyalgia rheumatica,** which causes pain and stiffness of the pelvic and shoulder muscles.
- **Give oral steroids immediately to prevent blindness.**
- **Temporal artery biopsy** confirms the diagnosis.

TENSION HEADACHE

- Tension headaches are typically bilateral and vise-like in character. Nonspecific symptoms such as poor concentration are common.
- Treat with analgesics and anxiety reduction.

THE WORST HEADACHE

- Subarachnoid hemorrhage typically presents as the worst headache in the patient's life.

Hematology and Oncology

ANEMIA

- **Iron deficiency is the #1 cause of anemia worldwide.** The #1 cause of iron deficiency in the U.S. is blood loss, particularly **GI bleeding.**
- Iron deficiency causes a **microcytic, hypochromic anemia.** A **serum ferritin $<$20 μg/L** is virtually pathognomonic. Serum iron will be low. Total iron binding capacity (TIBC) will be *high.* Absent iron stores in bone marrow is pathognomonic.
- Other causes of microcytic hypochromic anemia are thalassemia, lead poisoning, and sideroblastic anemia.
- Macrocytic anemia is commonly caused by vitamin B_{12} deficiency, folate deficiency, or reticulocytosis.

POLYCYTHEMIA VERA

- Polycythemia vera is the uncontrolled production of erythroid cells, which results in a high hematocrit. White blood cells and platelets may also be elevated.

- Patients look red and complain of itching.
- Splenomegaly and a **low erythropoietin level** should be present.
- Treat with **phlebotomy.**

Cardiology

ESSENTIAL HYPERTENSION

- Hypertension (HTN) is defined as blood pressure exceeding 140 mmHg systolic or 90 mmHg diastolic. **140/90 is the threshold.** Both systolic and diastolic HTN decrease life expectancy.
- **One high blood pressure reading does not make the diagnosis.** Bring patients back to recheck blood pressure.
- About 95% of HTN has no known cause (essential hypertension).
- Initial treatment includes diet, exercise, weight loss, abstinence from alcohol, and smoking cessation.
- **Diuretics and β-blockers reduce mortality** and are the first-line drugs.
- **Controlling HTN is the single most effective way to prevent stroke.**

SECONDARY HYPERTENSION

- In younger people, secondary HTN is more likely.
- **Oral contraceptives are the #1 cause of secondary HTN. Discontinue them.**
- Bilateral renal artery stenosis may cause abdominal bruits or be silent.
- Pheochromocytoma can cause episodic or chronic HTN. Elevated urine catecholamines and urine vanillylmandelic acid (VMA) are diagnostic.
- Coarctation of the aorta can present at any age. Typical signs include **upper body HTN** and **rib notching** on chest x-ray.

MALIGNANT HYPERTENSION

- Malignant HTN is a syndrome of very high blood pressure with end organ damage. Nephropathy or papilledema and encephalopathy may be seen.
- **Sodium nitroprusside** is the drug of choice to emergently lower high blood pressure.

Fluids and Electrolytes

BLOOD GASES

- Several arterial blood gases (ABGs) will be given. Each contains pH, Po_2, Pco_2, and HCO_3^-.
- Look at pH first. **pH defines acidosis vs. alkalosis.**
- Next, look at HCO_3^-. Low pH and low HCO_3^- is metabolic acidosis. High pH and high HCO_3^- is metabolic alkalosis. **If the HCO_3^- is normal or goes opposite the pH, then the primary disorder is probably respiratory.** Rarely, it will be a mixed disorder.
- Aspirin overdose (salicylism) causes respiratory alkalosis with metabolic acidosis. Patients may experience **tinnitus,** vomiting, and mental status changes. Treatment includes IV bicarbonate to **alkalinize the urine.**
- A few **causes of metabolic alkalosis are worth memorizing.** These include diuretics, vomiting, volume contraction, antacid abuse, and hyperaldosteronism.

HYPERCALCEMIA

- Cancer, hyperparathyroidism, and sarcoidosis are the main causes of hypercalcemia.
- **Multiple myeloma causes hypercalcemia.** Classic findings include a monoclonal spike on serum protein electrophoresis (SPEP) and punched-out lytic bone lesions on x-ray.
- Sarcoidosis occurs in younger adults and usually affects the lungs. Classic findings include **bilateral hilar lymphadenopathy** and noncaseating granulomas.
- Treat hypercalcemia with **saline and furosemide** (*not* thiazide diuretics).

Endocrinology

THYROID DISEASE

- Both hyper- and hypothyroidism cause weakness, fatigue, and menstrual irregularities.
- Hyperthyroidism causes tachycardia, tachyarrhythmias, and tremor.
- Hypothyroidism causes bradycardia, **hypertension,** and edema.
- **Free T_4** is the best indicator of thyroid state, but **free thyroxine index (FTI)** is more commonly used. A thyroid panel typically contains FTI, total T_4, and T_3 resin uptake. Usually all thyroid indices are high in hyperthyroidism and low in hypothyroidism.
- Serum TSH distinguishes primary vs. secondary disease.
    - In hyperthyroidism (defined by a **high FTI**), a low TSH means primary disease because the thyroid is hyperfunctioning on its own. A high TSH means the thyroid is responding normally to a secondary disease process.
    - In hypothyroidism (defined by a **low FTI**), a low TSH means the thyroid is responding normally to a secondary disease. A high TSH means primary disease.
- **Graves' disease** (diffuse toxic goiter) is the #1 cause of hyperthyroidism in the U.S. It is familial and most common in **young women. Antibodies against TSH receptors** stimulate thyroid hyperfunction. Treat with propranolol and ablate the thyroid with radioactive iodine.
- The #1 cause of hypothyroidism in the U.S. is **Hashimoto's thyroiditis.** Hashimoto's thyroiditis is most common in middle-aged women with goiter. **Anti-thyroglobulin and anti-mitochondrial antibodies** are seen. Lymphocytic infiltration is prominent. Treat with levothyroxine.
- Worldwide, the #1 cause of goiter is iodine deficiency.

HYPERALDOSTERONISM

- Aldosterone signals the kidneys to retain Na^+ and excrete K^+. Therefore, hyperaldosteronism leads to **high Na^+** and **low K^+.**

- In addition, **metabolic alkalosis** and **hypertension** are typical.

ADDISON'S DISEASE

- Addison's disease is adrenal cortex insufficiency. Hypoaldosteronism leads to **hyponatremia, hyperkalemia, and hypotension.**
- The diagnosis is made by finding **low serum cortisol** in the presence of **high ACTH.**
- In *pituitary* failure, ACTH is low but aldosterone is normal. Aldosterone is independent of the pituitary.

ANTIDIURETIC HORMONE

- Antidiuretic hormone (ADH) is also called vasopressin.
- SIADH, the syndrome of inappropriate ADH secretion, causes **euvolemic hyponatremia.** SIADH does not cause hypertension or edema.
  - **Urine osmolarity will be high,** even with a fluid challenge. If it is normal or low, think psychogenic polydipsia.
  - **Small cell lung cancer** is an important cause of SIADH.
- Diabetes insipidus causes **extreme polyuria and polydipsia** due to insufficient ADH.
  - Urine will be dilute.
  - Hypernatremia may occur.

PITUITARY TUMOR

- **Prolactinoma** is the #1 pituitary tumor. It presents with amenorrhea and sometimes galactorrhea. **Bromocriptine** is the initial treatment.
- If the tumor is calcified, it is a craniopharyngioma.

DIABETES MELLITUS

- Diabetes mellitus typically presents with polydipsia, polyuria, and hyperglycemia.
- In Type I diabetes (insulin-dependent diabetes), patients *die* without insulin. Type I diabetics are usually juveniles.

Antibodies against β islet cells in the pancreas are a hallmark.

- Type II diabetes (non–insulin-dependent diabetes) is far more common and typically presents in late adulthood. Obesity, hypertension, and atherosclerosis are common findings. Many Type II patients also take insulin.
- **A fasting serum glucose >140 mg/dL is diagnostic.**

DIABETIC COMA

Ketoacidosis	*Non-ketotic Hyperglycemic Coma*
Hyperglycemia present	Hyperglycemia present
Urinary **ketones present**	Urinary **ketones absent**
Usually patient is **Type I diabetic**	Usually patient is **Type II diabetic**
Treated with hydration and insulin	Treated with hydration and insulin
Frequently reversible	Frequently fatal

Gastroenterology

GASTROESOPHAGEAL REFLUX

- Reflux is diagnosed clinically. Heartburn is the hallmark.
- The #1 cause of reflux is intermittent relaxation of the lower esophageal sphincter.
- **Endoscopy** is the study of choice but is done only for severe or persistent disease.
    - **Barrett's esophagus** can give rise to adenocarcinoma. Manage Barrett's esophagus with endoscopy and biopsy every 2 years.
    - Peptic strictures must also be biopsied.
- The initial treatment includes diet changes, antacids, and H_2-blockers or omeprazole.

PANCREATITIS

- **Alcohol** and **gallstones** are the leading causes of both acute and chronic pancreatitis. Hypercalcemia and hypertriglyceridemia are other important causes.

- Acute pancreatitis presents with the **abrupt onset of steady and severe epigastric pain that often radiates to the back.** Usually there is **no guarding or rebound.**
  - Serum **amylase** rises before lipase, so amylase levels are checked in the emergency room.
  - **Hypocalcemia** correlates with a poor prognosis.

& hypoxia & metabolic acidosis

MALABSORPTION

- Severe malabsorption leads to foul, greasy stools which **stain positively for fat.**
- A positive **fecal D-xylose test** indicates intestinal disease (versus pancreatic insufficiency).
- Celiac sprue (gluten-sensitive enteropathy) is diagnosed by biopsy. The gluten-containing foods wheat, barley, and rye are removed from the diet.
- **Whipple's disease** is a systemic infection occurring in middle-aged males. In addition to malabsorption, fever, arthritis, and CNS manifestations are typical.
- Lactase deficiency causes diarrhea, intestinal cramps, and flatulence. Treat by removing dairy products from the diet.

HEMOCHROMATOSIS

- In hemochromatosis, iron-containing hemosiderin accumulates in the **liver, heart, and pancreas.** The term **bronze diabetes** comes from the diabetes mellitus and skin discoloration seen in late disease.
- Patients are usually older men.
- Cirrhosis and hepatocellular carcinoma may develop.
- High iron stores in a liver biopsy are diagnostic.
- Treat with deferoxamine and phlebotomy.

WILSON'S DISEASE

- Wilson's disease (hepatolenticular degeneration) is characterized by excessive copper storage in the **liver** and **brain.** It is rare.
- Patients develop cirrhosis, psychiatric problems, and tremor.

- A **low ceruloplasmin level** in the presence of elevated liver copper is diagnostic.
- Brownish gray or gold **Kayser-Fleischer rings** in the corneas are pathognomonic.

Infectious Disease

ANTIBIOTIC PROPHYLAXIS

- Congenital heart disease and serious valve disease require prophylactic antibiotics.
  - Give amoxicillin or penicillin 6 hours before and 6 hours after teeth cleaning, dental work, and throat surgery.
  - Give ampicillin and gentamicin for GI and GU procedures, including endoscopy.
- Tuberculosis prophylaxis is given to close contacts of patients with active tuberculosis and to people with a positive tuberculin skin test (PPD). Treat HIV patients if the PPD is >5 mm induration; other sick people if the PPD is >10 mm; and healthy people under age 35 if the PPD is >15 mm. Healthy people over 35 are not treated unless they are a close contact.
  - **Isoniazid alone** is used if the chest x-ray is negative.
  - Isoniazid may cause **hepatitis** and peripheral neuropathy. **Pyridoxine** (vitamin B_6) prevents isoniazid-induced neuropathy.

PNEUMONIA

- ***Streptococcus pneumoniae*** is the #1 cause of community-acquired pneumonia overall in patients older than 7.
- Among **teenagers and young adults, *Mycoplasma pneumoniae*** is the #1 cause. The cold agglutinin test is typically positive in *Mycoplasma* disease.
- Erythromycin is still the *empiric* treatment of choice for community-acquired pneumonia.

INFECTIOUS MONONUCLEOSIS

- Infectious mononucleosis is caused by Epstein-Barr virus. The classic symptoms are sore throat, lymphadenopathy, and hepatosplenomegaly.
- Lab findings include **positive heterophil antibody tests** such as the Monospot and lymphocytosis with **atypical lymphocytes.**
- **Ampicillin causes rash** in patients with infectious mononucleosis. Do not give it.
- **Splenic rupture** and hepatitis can occur.

URINARY TRACT INFECTION

- *E. coli* remains the #1 cause of UTI.
- Recurrent UTI requires a work-up for stones, obstruction, reflux, or other GU disease. In kids, **vesicoureteral reflux** is the #1 cause of recurrent UTI.
- Women with >3 UTIs per year are given prophylactic antibiotics nightly or after sexual intercourse.

MICROBIOLOGY

Infection Setting	*Bug To Remember*
Boils, furuncles, and carbuncles	*Staph aureus*
Osteomyelitis	*Staph aureus*
Surgical wound	*Staph aureus*
IV drug user with heart murmur	*Staph aureus*
Burn infection	*Pseudomonas*
Red ear canal or ear	*Pseudomonas*
Nail injury through shoe	*Pseudomonas*
Cat or dog bite	*Pasteurella*
Cellulitis	Group A *Strep, Staph aureus*
Splenectomy	*S. pneumoniae, H. influenzae, N. meningitidis*
Traveler's diarrhea	*E. coli*
Pericarditis	Coxsackie B virus

Lab Test Interpretation

- For the USMLE Step 2, basic lab knowledge usually suffices. Keep in mind that each test booklet contains complete tables of normal lab values.

PULMONARY FUNCTION TESTS

- Obstructive lung disease is characterized by a **low FEV_1** and low FEV_1/FVC ratio. FVC will be normal or low.
  - **Total lung capacity will be normal or high.**
  - COPD and asthma are the classic obstructive diseases.
- Restrictive lung disease is characterized by **low total lung capacity.** Tidal volume may be normal.
  - FEV_1 and FVC may be decreased, but the lung volumes make the diagnosis.
  - Examples of restrictive lung disease include lung resection, pulmonary infiltrates, and diaphragm movement disorders such as phrenic nerve paralysis.

LIVER FUNCTION TESTS

- Alkaline phosphatase is produced in bile ducts, bones, and placentas. For most questions, an elevated alkaline phosphatase with normal AST and ALT means **obstruction of the bile ducts** or **bone metastases.** Other possibilities are pregnancy and older age.
- If AST and ALT are both >250 IU/L, infectious hepatitis is the leading diagnosis.
- If AST is elevated much more than ALT, alcoholic liver injury is the most likely diagnosis.
- The liver conjugates bilirubin. A high unconjugated bilirubin (indirect or insoluble bilirubin) indicates **intravascular hemolysis** or failure of the liver to take up bilirubin as in Gilbert's syndrome.

ELECTROLYTES

- A BUN/creatinine ratio greater than 20:1 usually means dehydration.

Toxicology

Toxin	*Syndrome*	*Antidote*
Acetaminophen	**Hepatic necrosis**	**N-acetylcysteine**
Opioids	Respiratory depression, pinpoint pupils	Naloxone
Organophosphates	Muscarinic agonism effects	Pralidoxime, atropine
Heparin	Bleeding	Protamine
Warfarin	Bleeding	Vitamin K

Advanced Life Support for the USMLE Step 2, by Flynn et al.
Lippincott–Raven Publishers © 1997.

CHAPTER 7

Neurology and Neurosurgery

Ketan R. Bulsara

Study Hints

- Lesion localization and common neurologic disorders are high yield.
- Use the schematic in Figure 7-1 to group these disorders.

Muscle

POLYMYOSITIS

- Polymyositis is a systemic disorder whose principal finding is proximal muscle weakness.
- **Extraocular muscles are not affected.**
- **Creatine phosphokinase (CPK) is elevated.** The erythrocyte sedimentation rate (ESR) may be normal or elevated.
- Muscle biopsy confirms the diagnosis.

DERMATOMYOSITIS

- Dermatomyositis is polymyositis with skin manifestations.
- Look for **purple or heliotropic (reddish-purple) upper eyelids.**
- The risk of **cancer** is greater with dermatomyositis.

Categories of Neurologic Dysfunction
Brain dysfunction
• Cognition deficits
• Typically unilateral motor or sensory deficits
Spinal cord dysfunction
• Sensory levels
• Symmetric distal weakness
• Incontinence
• Hyperreflexia and clonus
• Positive Babinski
Peripheral nerve dysfunction
• Asymmetric distal weakness
• Atrophy and fasciculations
• Hyporeflexia
Muscle dysfunction
• Symmetric proximal weakness

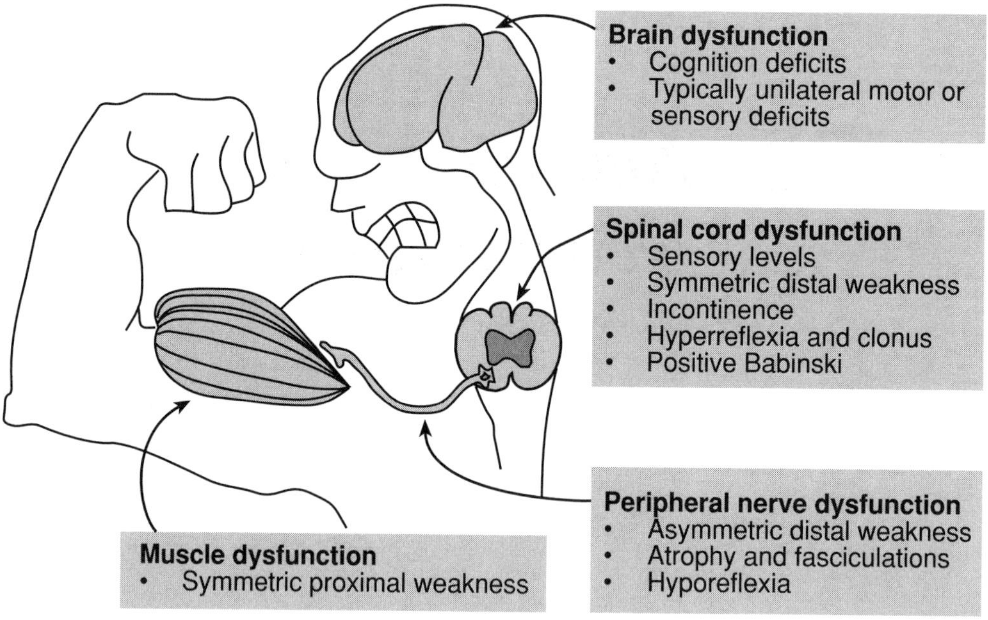

Figure 7-1

DUCHENNE MUSCULAR DYSTROPHY

- Duchenne is the most common muscular dystrophy. It presents in childhood.
- It is an X-linked **absence of dystrophin.**
- Look for **large calves** caused by pseudohypertrophy.
- Death usually occurs by age 20.

Neuromuscular Junction

MYASTHENIA GRAVIS

- **Autoantibodies block acetylcholine receptors.**
- **Muscles fatigue quickly** (vs. Lambert-Eaton).
- **Extraocular muscles are affected** (vs. Lambert-Eaton).
- Acetylcholinesterase inhibitors such as edrophonium and neostigmine result in dramatic improvement.
- **Thymectomy** helps most patients.

- Plasmapheresis and immunosuppressive agents are also used.

LAMBERT-EATON SYNDROME

- Serum antibodies decrease acetylcholine release at the neuromuscular junction by blocking voltage-gated calcium channels.
- **Muscles get stronger with repeated movement** because acetylcholine accumulates.
- **Extraocular muscles are usually not affected,** although ptosis may be present.
- Severe autonomic dysfunction may be present.
- **Small cell carcinoma** of the lung is commonly associated.
- Surgical treatment consists of tumor resection.

BOTULISM

- The toxin may be found in **bulging cans,** especially home-canned foods. Honey is the classic source for infant botulism.
- **Constipation** is a common complaint.
- Within 48 hours following ingestion, extraocular muscle paralysis occurs. **Flaccid paralysis** and respiratory failure follow.
- Infants present with constipation, a weak cry and smile, and hypotonia with poor head control. A symmetric, descending paralysis may also be present.
- Mental status remains intact.

Peripheral Nerve

AIDS NEUROPATHY

- AIDS patients sometimes develop foot paresthesias and decreased vibratory and light touch sensation.
- AZT and ddI are common iatrogenic causes.

CARPAL TUNNEL SYNDROME

- Repetitive trauma is the most common cause.
- **Females** are more commonly affected.

- **Median nerve entrapment** at the wrist by the flexor retinaculum ligament leads to painful paresthesias.
- Signs include **thenar atrophy** and a weak grip. Clinical tests that trigger symptoms include 30–60 seconds of wrist flexion **(Phalen's test)** and percussing over the flexor retinaculum ligament **(Tinel's test).**
- Medical management includes rest, NSAIDs, wrist splints, and steroid injections.
- Complete surgical division of the flexor retinaculum is another option.

LUMBAR DISC HERNIATION

- The disc that most commonly herniates is **L5-S1.**
- Symptoms include **dermatomal pain** over the lower extremity with sensory changes.
- The **straight leg raising test** exacerbates symptoms.
- Nonsurgical management includes rest and NSAIDs.
- Surgical management includes lumbar laminectomy with discectomy.

DIABETIC NEUROPATHY

- Diabetes causes a distal **sensory polyneuropathy. Autonomic neuropathy** may also be present.
- Symptoms and signs include pain, paresthesias, and **loss of distal vibration sense.**
- The **symmetric** extremity involvement differentiates diabetic neuropathy from most other neuropathies.
- Treat by **tightly controlling blood glucose levels.**
- Amitriptyline or desipramine may relieve symptoms.

Spinal Cord

BROWN-SÉQUARD SYNDROME

- **Unilateral hemisection** of the spinal cord causes **ipsilateral motor weakness** or paralysis with loss of tactile and vibratory sensation.

- Patients also lose **contralateral** pain and temperature sensation.

SYRINGOMYELIA

- A **cystic cavity** forms within the spinal cord.
- The communicating type is associated with the mild cerebellar herniation of Chiari I malformations.
- The noncommunicating type is associated with trauma.
- The Brown-Séquard syndrome may occur.
- Surgical treatments include shunts and cyst aspiration.

Brainstem and Cortex

TRANSIENT ISCHEMIC ATTACKS

- Emboli from the **carotid artery** can cause **amaurosis fugax,** which is a transient ipsilateral monocular blindness.
- **Vertebral artery** emboli may present with brain stem findings such as **diplopia, dysarthria, or homonymous hemianopsia.**
- Angiography is the gold standard for evaluation of carotid stenosis.
- Medical management includes **anticoagulation.**
- Treat severe carotid disease with **carotid endarterectomy.**

STROKES

- **Vasculopathies** and **coagulopathies** cause strokes.
- **Lacunar infarcts** are small-vessel thrombotic events. Hypertensive patients are most vulnerable.
- The most effective preventive measure is **treating hypertension.**

HYDROCEPHALUS

- **Communicating** hydrocephalus results from inadequate CSF reabsorption.
- **Noncommunicating** hydrocephalus results from an obstruction of CSF flow within the ventricular system.

- Common symptoms and signs include headache, nausea, and vomiting.
- The surgical management is CSF shunting.

EPIDURAL HEMATOMA

- **The classic patient briefly loses consciousness, then is lucid for several hours before losing consciousness again.**
- Typically, a temporoparietal skull fracture cuts the **middle meningeal artery.**
- CT scans reveal **biconvex densities** adjacent to the skull that may cross the midline.
- Most cases are neurosurgical emergencies. Operate quickly to avoid uncal or cerebellar herniation.

ACUTE SUBDURAL HEMATOMA

- **Bridging veins** are torn by cerebral acceleration-deceleration during violent head motion.
- Presentations vary.
- CT scans reveal **crescent-shaped densities** adjacent to the skull that never cross the midline.
- Surgical decompression is indicated if the patient is neurologically unstable or the hematoma is greater than 1 cm.

SUBARACHNOID HEMORRHAGE

- Patients classically present with **"the worst headache ever."**
- **Mental status may be altered.**
- Sterile meningitis characterized by photophobia, fever, and stiff neck may occur.
- Confirm the diagnosis with a CT scan or lumbar puncture.
- Use cerebral **angiograms** to locate the lesion.
- **Trauma is the #1 cause.** Aneurysm rupture is the #2 cause.
- Treat with surgical clip ligation of any operable aneurysms.

Other Commonly Tested Disorders

MULTIPLE SCLEROSIS

- Multiple sclerosis typically presents between ages **20 and 40.**
- **Females** are more commonly affected.
- Common complaints include **diplopia,** decreased visual acuity, spastic paraparesis, and incontinence.
- Multiple sclerosis may present with **optic neuritis.**
- **Multiple diffuse plaques** result from demyelination of white matter.
- Increased CSF IgG and oligoclonal bands may be present.
- MRI is the imaging modality of choice.
- Treatment is supportive.
- Exacerbations and remissions are typical.

AMYOTROPHIC LATERAL SCLEROSIS

- Onset typically occurs **after age 40.**
- **Degeneration of both upper and lower motor neurons occurs.**
- Atrophy, **fasciculations,** and spasticity may be present.
- Voluntary muscles of the eye and sphincter are spared.
- Mental status remains intact.
- Death usually occurs within 5 years of onset.

GUILLAIN-BARRÉ SYNDROME

- **Viral upper respiratory infections** or **immunizations** usually precede the syndrome by a few days.
- Patients present with an **ascending peripheral paralysis** due to focal segmental demyelination.
- Complications include respiratory failure.
- Recovery may take months. Early **plasmapheresis** may hasten recovery.

COCAINE

- Cocaine blocks the reuptake of norepinephrine, which leads to euphoria, dilated pupils, and hypertension.
- Cocaine can cause **seizures, brain hemorrhages, and strokes.**

Advanced Life Support for the USMLE Step 2, by Flynn et al.
Lippincott–Raven Publishers © 1997.

CHAPTER 8

Surgery

Albert S. Y. Chang and Bryan J. Krol

Study Hints

- Critical care physiology is high yield.
- Penetrating trauma to the chest is high yield.
- The differential diagnosis of the acute abdomen is high yield.
- Indications for surgery are high yield.
- Surgical procedures are low yield.
- Cancer staging is very low yield.

Trauma

- Always remember **ABC-IV. A**irway → **B**reathing → **C**irculation → IV access. When in doubt, **intubate.** If intubation is not possible, perform a cricothyrotomy.
- Order cervical spine, chest, and pelvic x-rays for all trauma cases.
- Unstable patients typically undergo surgery, intubation, or other dramatic interventions. *Unstable* means hypotensive, severely bleeding, losing the airway, in a life-threatening arrhythmia, or otherwise in danger of dying soon.

HEAD TRAUMA

- Skull fractures are evaluated with CT scans.

- Depressed skull fractures should be surgically elevated if the depression exceeds 1 cm.
- Basilar skull fractures cause CSF leakage and a positive Battle's sign, which is bruising over the mastoid behind the ear. Blood may be seen behind the eardrums.
- **A penetrating wound to zone 2 of the neck,** the area between the clavicle and lower mandible, should be **surgically explored after intubation.**

CNS TRAUMA

- Treat blunt spinal cord trauma with **steroids.**
- Rule out intracranial hemorrhage with CT scans. If the CT is negative, perform a lumbar puncture.
- Cross-table lateral cervical spine films are mandatory.

THORACIC TRAUMA

- Myocardial contusion can lead to arrhythmias, CHF, and ventricular aneurysms.
- Cardiac tamponade leads to distended neck veins, decreased pulse pressure, muffled heart sounds, and decreased voltage on ECG. **Echocardiograms** confirm the diagnosis. With unstable patients, proceed directly to **pericardiocentesis** without doing an echocardiogram.
- Large or tension pneumothoraces cause hypotension, tracheal deviation, decreased breath sounds, and distended neck veins. Treat with thoracostomy.
- Hemothorax also causes hypotension and tracheal deviation, but breath sounds will be normal and the neck veins will be collapsed.
- Small pneumothoraces should be followed by chest x-ray every 24 hours.
- **Flail chest** is caused by ribs breaking in two or more spots, allowing paradoxical movement of the chest wall.
- A bullet entering the circulation can embolize.

ABDOMINAL TRAUMA

- If the patient is unstable, **perform diagnostic peritoneal lavage.** Place a nasogastric tube and empty the bladder first.
- If the patient is stable, order a CT scan of the abdomen and pelvis.

- **Splenectomy is warranted in splenic rupture.** Always vaccinate against *Streptococcus pneumoniae, Neisseria meningitidis,* and *Hemophilus influenzae B.*
- A stable pelvic hematoma with pelvic fracture **should not be explored.**
- Pelvic fractures are unstable if the main pelvic ring has two breaks. Treat with pneumatic trousers, external or internal fixation, and embolization of any bleeding vessels.

CHOKING

- Leave choking patients alone if they can speak, breathe, or cough. Otherwise, use abdominal thrusts. If that fails, perform a cricothyrotomy.

ENVIRONMENTAL TRAUMA

- Figure 8-1 illustrates some types of environmental trauma.

SHOCK

- Shock leads to mottled skin, hypotension, hypoperfusion, and altered mental status.
- **Use invasive hemodynamic monitoring.**

Type of Shock	*CO*	*PCWP*	*PVR*	*Notes*
Cardiogenic	Low	High	High	Low SvO_2
Hypovolemic	Low	Low	High	Low SvO_2
Neurogenic	Low	Low	Low	Low SvO_2
Septic	High	Low	Low	High SvO_2, high SaO_2

CO, cardiac output; *PCWP,* pulmonary capillary wedge pressure; *PVR,* peripheral vascular resistance; *SvO_2,* systemic venous oxygen saturation; *SaO_2,* systemic arterial oxygen saturation.

VENTILATORS

- Intubation is indicated in cases of refractory hypoxemia, failure to ventilate (rising CO_2), inability to protect the airway, and **impending doom.**
- Positive end expiratory pressure (PEEP) prevents atelectasis.
- In weaning a patient from a ventilator, **reduce FIO_2 first,** then respiratory rate, then PEEP (down to 5 cm H_2O), and finally pressure support.
- Always change just one ventilator setting at a time.

Environmental Trauma

Burns

- Perform escharotomy to prevent nerve entrapment or ventilatory restriction.
- Treat with fluids, respiratory monitoring, and topical silver products. **Do not use steroids**.
- *Psuedomonas* commonly infects burns.

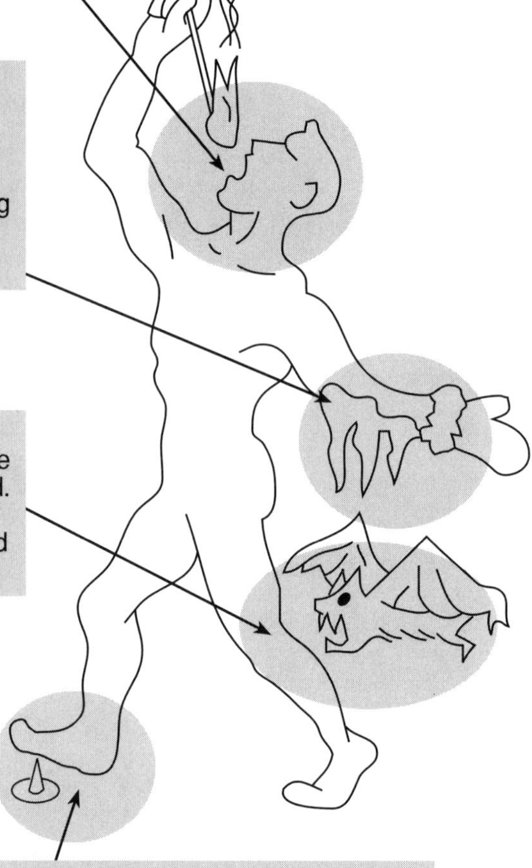

Hypothermic injury

- Hypothermia can cause arrhythmias, altered mental status, muscle rigidity, and respiratory or metabolic acidosis.
- Treat frostbite with rapid wet rewarming to no higher than 42° Celsius. Wait 2 weeks to debride.

Rabies prophylaxis

- If the biting animal can be captured, the animal should be monitored or sacrificed.
- If the animal is infected or cannot be captured, treat with rabies vaccine and rabies hyperimmune globulin.

Tetanus prophylaxis

- Patients who have had < 3 tetanus toxoid shots in their lives get tetanus toxoid for any wound. They also get tetanus hyperimmune globulin for dirty or severe wounds.
- Patients who have had ≥ 3 tetanus toxoid shots get toxoid for clean wounds if their last shot was > 10 years ago. They get toxoid for severe of dirty wounds if their last shot was > 5 years ago.

Figure 8-1

CRITICAL CARE DRUGS

- **Use epinephrine to treat anaphylaxis,** status asthmaticus, and asystole.
- Use furosemide to treat acute pulmonary edema and cerebral edema.
- Treat opioid toxicity with naloxone.
- Use dantrolene to treat malignant hyperthermia due to halothane or succinylcholine.
- Digoxin slows AV node conduction and increases contractility. Negative effects include bradycardia, nausea, vomiting, yellow vision, and arrhythmias.

Acute Abdomen

LOCALIZING INFLAMMATION

- Diaphragmatic lesions such as liver abscesses and perforated gastric ulcers may cause pain on top of the shoulders and in a necklace distribution (C4 nerve roots).
- Small intestine disease causes pain in the epigastric and umbilical regions.
- Large intestine disease causes pain in the hypogastric region.
- Biliary distention causes pain in the right subscapular region.
- The testicles descend from around the kidneys. Pain radiating to the testicles can be due to genitourinary disease or appendicitis.
- Suspect peptic ulcer disease in patients on steroids.

HISTORY

- **Syncope** suggests a grave situation such as perforated ulcer, acute pancreatitis, ruptured aortic aneurysm, or ruptured ectopic pregnancy.
- Vomiting can help distinguish between competing diagnoses.
  - **Bile-tinged vomit indicates colic or duodenal atresia.**
  - **Feculent vomit is pathognomonic for small bowel obstruction.**

Abdominal Pain

General
- **Small bowel obstruction** causes **bilious vomiting**, abdominal distention, constipation, and episodic pain with hyperactive and high-pitched bowel sounds. Late findings include tachycardia, hypotension, and fever.
- **Large bowel obstruction** causes gradually increasing pain, constipation, and abdominal distention.

Epigastric
- **Pancreatitis** causes severe steady focal pain of sudden onset with radiation to the back. Nausea, vomiting, anorexia, and decreased bowel sounds are frequent findings.
- **Abdominal aortic aneurysm rupture** causes upper abdominal pain, back pain, and hypovolemia or shock. A large **pulsatile mass** is classic.

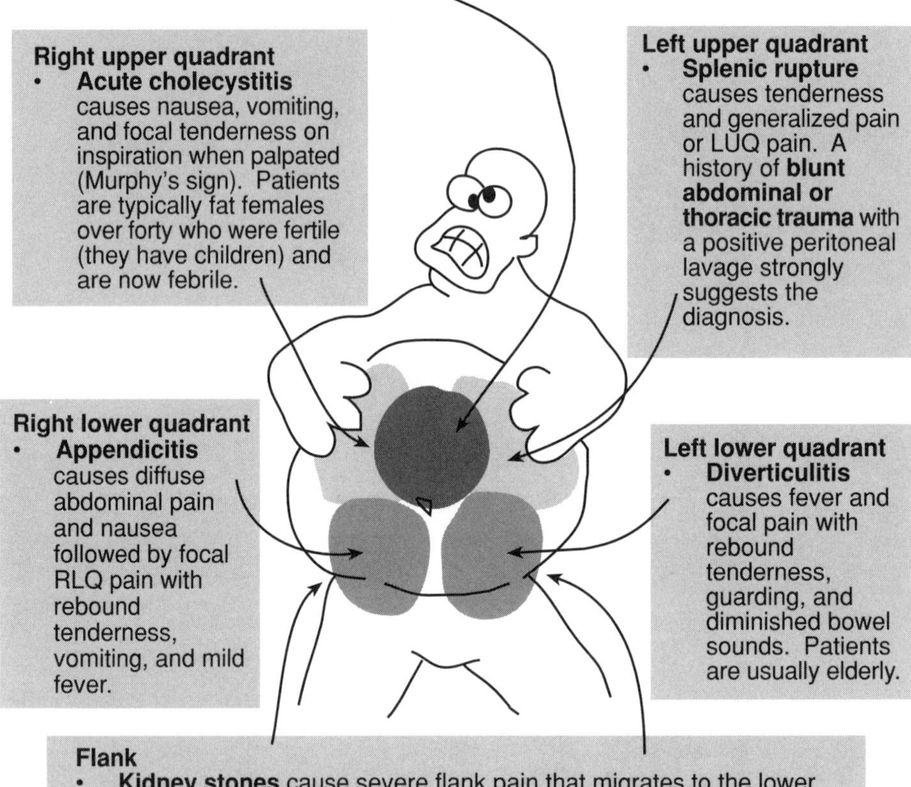
Right upper quadrant
• Acute cholecystitis causes nausea, vomiting, and focal tenderness on inspiration when palpated (Murphy's sign). Patients are typically fat females over forty who were fertile (they have children) and are now febrile.
Left upper quadrant
• Splenic rupture causes tenderness and generalized pain or LUQ pain. A history of blunt abdominal or thoracic trauma with a positive peritoneal lavage strongly suggests the diagnosis.
Right lower quadrant
• Appendicitis causes diffuse abdominal pain and nausea followed by focal RLQ pain with rebound tenderness, vomiting, and mild fever.
Left lower quadrant
• Diverticulitis causes fever and focal pain with rebound tenderness, guarding, and diminished bowel sounds. Patients are usually elderly.

Flank
- **Kidney stones** cause severe flank pain that migrates to the lower abdomen as the stones pass along the ureter. It is usually treated medically.
- **Pyelonephritis** causes flank pain with urinary frequency and urgency. It is treated medically.

Additional clues
- Severe shock implies bleeding or thrombosis.
- Rigidity implies inflammation.
- For all abdominal pain, rule out medical problems such as myocardial infarction and herpes zoster and reexamine the patient 2—3 hours later.

Figure 8-2

- Vomiting decreases the acid content of the stomach. Pain due to perforated peptic ulcer will decrease, and the vomiting will stop. Vomiting does not ease pain due to strangulated bowel or genitourinary disease. In these cases, vomiting will continue.

- Constant epigastric pain which worsens with eating suggests carcinoma or chronic gastric ulcer.
- **Pain a few hours after eating suggests duodenal ulcer.**

PHYSICAL EXAM

- If the patient is immobile, suspect peritonitis.
- If the pain increases when reclining and decreases when sitting up, suspect retroperitoneal disease.

Orthopedics

FRACTURES

- Fractures are covered in Chapter 9, the chapter on the glossy book.

TISSUE INJURIES

- Volkmann's contracture is contraction of the fingers or wrist due to vascular insufficiency. Severe injury to the elbow and improper tourniquet use are causes. Treat with immediate decompression.
- A felon is a pulp-space infection of the distal finger pad. Tension may impair blood supply. Treat with incision and drainage.
- A paronychia is an infection adjacent to the nail. Treat with incision and drainage.

Breast Disease

BREAST CANCER

- **The major risk factors are a personal history of breast cancer, female gender, age greater than 40, and a family**

history of breast cancer in a first degree relative. Minor risk factors include early menarche, late menopause, obesity, and low-dose radiation exposure.

- Cancerous masses are **usually unilateral and not movable.** Skin dimpling, nipple retraction, and axillary or supraclavicular lymphadenopathy may also be present.
- Nipple discharges are usually benign, the exception being bloody discharge with a mass.
- **Infiltrating ductal carcinoma** causes 70% of breast cancer. Other types of breast cancer include papillary carcinoma, medullary carcinoma, and Paget's disease, which is cancer with nipple and skin involvement.
- On mammography, malignant lesions typically have a spiculated or stellate appearance with *micro*calcifications.
- Any suspicious breast lesion should worked up by fine-needle aspiration or biopsy.
- Modified radical mastectomy and lumpectomy with axillary node dissection and adjuvant radiation therapy are **equally effective** for tumors less than 5 cm in size.
- Adjuvant endocrine therapy with **tamoxifen** is indicated for postmenopausal women with tumors that **express estrogen or progesterone receptors.**

FIBROADENOMA

- Fibroadenoma typically occurs in women in their **teens and twenties.**
- They are **solitary, encapsulated, freely movable masses.**
- **There is no increased risk for cancer.**
- If treatment is desired, do a lumpectomy.

FIBROCYSTIC CHANGE

- Fibrocystic change typically presents as painful bilateral breast nodularity in young or middle-aged women. The nodules often change with the menstrual cycle.
- Initial evaluation consists of observation over time or fine-needle aspiration of suspicious masses. Formal biopsy is necessary if aspiration does not reveal the green or dark amber fluid of simple cysts.

Lung Disease

LUNG CANCER

- Symptoms of bronchogenic carcinoma include **cough, weight loss, dyspnea, chest pain, and hemoptysis.**
- Additional symptom complexes include **Horner's syndrome** (ptosis, miosis, and anhidrosis), superior vena cava syndrome, and paraneoplastic syndromes such as Cushing's syndrome and SIADH.
- Small cell carcinoma represents 20% of all lung cancers and has a mean survival rate of 2–4 months. Treatment for small cell carcinoma is usually palliative.
- Non–small cell cancers have a better prognosis than small cell cancers.
  - **Squamous cell carcinomas arise centrally** in the chest.
  - **Adenocarcinomas usually arise peripherally** or diffusely throughout the chest.
  - Large cell or undifferentiated cancer usually arises **peripherally** in the chest.
- Resect non–small cell lung cancers *unless* there is a bloody pleural effusion, evidence of extensive local invasion into major nerves or blood vessels, or distant metastases.

BENIGN LUNG TUMORS

- Bronchial adenomas are located centrally and are highly vascularized. They are diagnosed by bronchoscopy.
- Hamartomas typically present in males over the age of 60 as peripheral lesions with **popcorn calcifications** seen on chest x-ray.

Vascular Surgery

CAROTID ARTERY STENOSIS

- Surgery is indicated for **patients with TIAs** (classically amaurosis fugax), **asymptomatic patients with >75% stenosis** of the carotid artery by arteriogram, and patients with good function after a stroke caused by carotid artery occlusion.

ABDOMINAL AORTIC ANEURYSM

- Approximately 95% of AAAs occur **below the renal arteries.** The inferior mesenteric artery is often occluded.
- AAA repair is indicated for any symptomatic patient and for any aneurysm >5 cm.
- AAA repair can lead to postoperative mesenteric ischemia.

PERIPHERAL VASCULAR DISEASE

- Findings include **shiny, hairless skin** with thickened toenails, pallor on elevation, redness on lowering, and diminished pulses and blood pressure in the lower extremities.
- Claudication alone is not an indication for surgery. Many patients can improve with nonsurgical therapies such as **smoking cessation.**
- Patients with rest pain, ischemic ulceration of the foot, or symptoms interfering with lifestyle are candidates for amputation.

DISSECTING AORTIC ANEURYSM

- Etiologies include **atherosclerosis, Marfan's syndrome, syphilis,** hypertension, trauma, and congenital heart defects.
- Patients typically present with **sudden severe pain radiating to the back.**
- Physical exam may reveal differing blood pressures in the upper extremities, hypotension, or diminished pulses and pressure in the lower extremities.
- Stabilize the patient and **induce hypotension** with nitroprusside and β-blockers.
- **Ascending aortic dissections and those involving the aortic arch require immediate surgery.**

- Descending aortic dissections can be treated medically with antihypertensives. Operate if hypertension continues or if the patient gets worse.

Urology

TESTICULAR DISEASE

- **Testicular torsion** is a surgical emergency. It typically presents as acute testicular pain in **10–20-year olds.** You have 4 hours to operate.
- Testicular cancers are the most common solid tumors in men 15–35 years old. All patients should undergo unilateral orchiectomy.
- Germ cell seminoma is the #1 primary testicular cancer. Treat with unilateral orchiectomy and radiation. The cure rate is high.
- A hydrocele is a cystic enlargement of the tunica vaginalis. It **transilluminates.** An inguinal hernia will not transilluminate. Aspiration of a hydrocele yields clear fluid. Treat surgically.
- A varicocele is a varicosity of the pampiniform venous plexus. It can lead to aching, infertility, and a dragging sensation.

URINARY TRACT DISEASE

- Renal cell carcinoma presents with a flank mass, hematuria, and abdominal pain.
- Transitional cell carcinoma is the most common bladder cancer. It is associated with smoking and aniline dyes.

Head Surgery

VERTIGO

- Meniere's syndrome is characterized by episodic vertigo with **unilateral tinnitus and deafness.**

- Positional vertigo is the most common vertigo disorder. The vertigo follows a change in position of the head, lasts less than 1 minute, involves **nystagmus,** and usually resolves spontaneously. Unlike Meniere's syndrome, there is no tinnitus or deafness.

FACIAL DISEASE

- Trigeminal neuralgia causes intense unilateral pain, usually in the distribution of CN V_2. Treat with carbamazepine or surgery.
- Sinusitis is diagnosed by x-rays or CT scan. Air-fluid levels and mucosal thickening are diagnostic. Treat acute infectious sinusitis with amoxicillin or amoxicillin/clavulanate. Chronic sinusitis is often caused by **sinus ostia obstruction.** Surgery may be required. Treating sinusitis is important because infection may extend into the frontal lobes or orbits.
- **Postoperative parotiditis** is usually caused by *Staphylococcus aureus.* It has a **20% mortality rate.**

CANCERS

- Acoustic neuromas arise in CN VIII at the cerebellopontine angle. Like Meniere's syndrome, there is unilateral hearing loss and tinnitus. Usually, however, the patient experiences chronic imbalance rather than vertigo.
- Nasopharyngeal cancer occurs in young adults. It is associated with the Epstein-Barr virus. Treat with radiation therapy and radical neck dissection if nodes are palpable.
- Laryngeal cancer causes persistent hoarseness. 90% are squamous cell carcinomas. **Heavy smokers or drinkers** account for 90% of patients. Treat with surgery or radiation.
- Parotid tumors are typically **benign.** Pleomorphic (mixed) tumors are most common.
- Thyroid cancers are more common in **women.** Patients are usually **euthyroid.**
  - **Papillary carcinoma** is the #1 thyroid cancer. Patients often have enlarged cervical lymph nodes.
  - Medullary carcinomas cause elevated calcitonin levels. They are associated with MEN-II and MEN-III.

- Cold nodules on nuclear scan should be biopsied.
- Treat with surgery, making sure to avoid the recurrent laryngeal nerve and leave at least one parathyroid gland. Postoperative radioactive iodine, direct radiotherapy, and thyroid hormone replacement are also used.

- Primary hyperparathyroidism is usually due to a single parathyroid adenoma. It causes **hypercalcemia, hypophosphatemia,** and increased urinary calcium. The diagnostic study of choice and treatment of choice are both neck exploration and excision of the adenoma. No studies need be done prior to exploration.

Advanced Life Support for the USMLE Step 2, by Flynn et al.
Lippincott–Raven Publishers © 1997.

CHAPTER 9

Return of the Glossy Book

Matt Flynn

Study Hints

- The fourth and last test booklet contains high-quality photographs. It can cause a lot of pain for the unprepared, but the good news is there just aren't that many things that photograph well.
- Dermatology is very high yield.
- Retinal pathology is high yield, but the clinical description usually gives away the disease.
- Radiology is high yield.
- Gram stains are high yield.
- The USMLE Step 2 authors are more refined than their Step 1 counterparts. You will not see many (if any) gross pathology specimens after lunch on the USMLE Step 2.

Lab Tests

GRAM STAINS

- Gram stains are infrequent, but they are easy points.
- Gram-positives are dark blue (remember **B+**).
  - Cocci in clusters are *Staphylococcus aureus.*

- Cocci in pairs and chains are *Streptococcus pneumoniae.*
- There are other *Staph* and *Strep* species, but they are rarely the answer.

- Gram-negatives are red. **If you are not sure of the color, it is gram-negative.**
  - Tiny rods are *Hemophilus influenzae.*
  - If there are gram-negative diplococci, the answer depends on location.

    Lungs: *Moraxella catarrhalis*
    CSF: *Neisseria meningitidis*
    Urethra: *Neisseria gonorrhea*
    Septic joint: *Neisseria gonorrhea*

PERIPHERAL SMEARS

- Blood smears appear exclusively in the glossy book. Usually the smear is straightforward, although the question may be hard. Look for classic findings such as sickled cells, spherocytes, or microcytic hypochromic cells.

ELECTROCARDIOGRAMS

- ECGs may appear in any book. Typically there are few. Quality is poor.
- Look for ischemia and infarction, manifested by T wave inversion, ST segment depression or elevation, and Q waves.
- Look for stark arrhythmias such as wide-complex ventricular tachycardia.

X-Rays

GENERAL RADIOLOGY

- X-rays can appear anywhere, but most are in the glossy book. The pictures are small, so only obvious findings will be tested.

- Bilateral hilar lymphadenopathy is usually sarcoidosis.
- A large opaque area on chest x-ray is usually lobar pneumonia.
- In a pneumothorax, lung vessels stop abruptly before reaching the chest wall. Do not miss the lung edge with clear space outside of it.
- The solitary lung nodule is a classic diagnostic challenge. **Compare with old films first.** If it is not growing, it is probably benign. Then get a CT scan before performing a transthoracic needle biopsy.
- Ring-enhancing lesions on contrast CT scans are difficult to diagnose. Patients with infections (e.g., sinusitis) typically have an **abscess.** AIDS patients commonly have **toxoplasmosis.** Other possibilities include tumor, infarction, and resolving bleed.

ORTHOPEDICS (Fig. 9-1)

- Orthopedics questions often give x-rays and ask for the best treatment.
- X-rays taken soon after a fracture may not reveal the break. Immobilize suspicious wrists and ankles, and repeat the x-rays in a week or later.
- Growth plates in children can look like fractures. Watch for the child with a normal arm or wrist.
- Clavicle fractures in **adults** should be treated with a **supporting sling.**
- Humerus fractures can cause injury to the radial nerve leading to wrist drop. They are treated with open or closed reduction and fixation.
- Simple closed femur fractures are treated with **traction only.**

Pores and Sores

- Dermatologists love to take photos almost as much as they like writing exam questions. If there had been any more skin in the recent glossy books, they would have had to serve them in a plain brown wrapper.

Orthopedics

Infancy and childhood

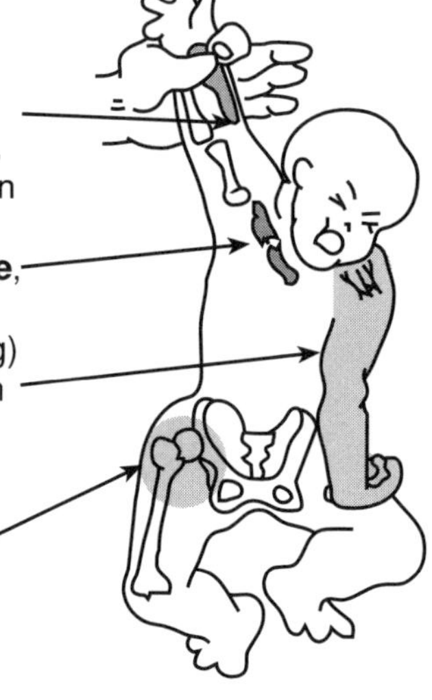

Nursemaid's elbow	Radial head subluxation in small child grabbed by hand, treated with manual reduction (i.e., supination)
Clavicle fracture	**Most common birth fracture**, heals without treatment in infants (treat adults with sling)
Erb-Duchenne palsy	Brachial plexus (C5-C6) birth injury causes **"waiter's tip"** posture (adduction and pronation of arm)
Congenital hip dislocation	"Click" with abduction on physical exam, treated with harness or double diapers

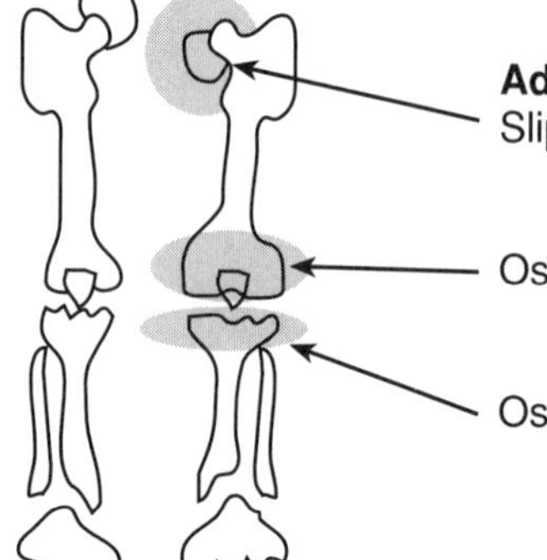

Adolescence

Slipped capital femoral epiphysis	Presents as painful hip or knee in **obese adolescent boys**, requires surgical fixation
Osteosarcoma	**The most common bone tumor in children**, two thirds occur around the knees
Osgood-Schlatter	Tibial tubercle inflammation (apophysitis), treated symptomatically

Adults

Femoral neck fracture	**Thin old women**, presents as groin pain or inability to lift leg, high risk of **avascular necrosis**, treat with **internal (open) fixation**, may require total hip arthroplasty in women > 70 years old
Colles' fracture	**"Fall on outstretched hand,"** the #1 wrist fracture (distal radius), treated with closed reduction and splinting
Scaphoid fracture	Most common carpal bone fracture, presents as **"snuffbox" tenderness**, high risk of **avascular necrosis**, treated with immobilization, normal initial radiographs should be repeated in 3 weeks

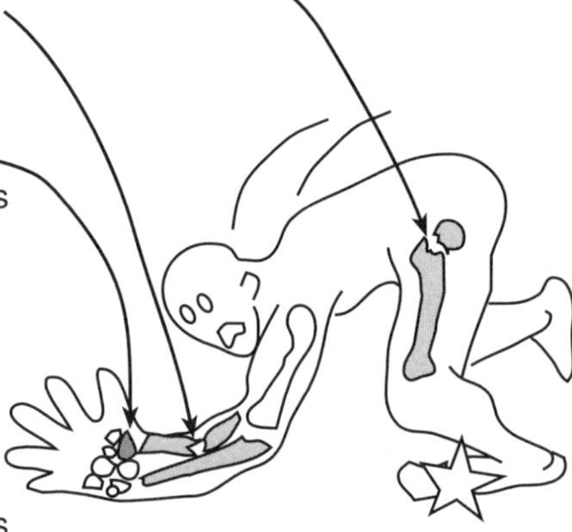

Figure 9-1

TOP DIAGNOSES

Top Diagnosis	*Identification and Important Facts*
Acne vulgaris	Use **tretinoin cream** (Retin-A) if benzoyl peroxide fails. Topical clindamycin or oral tetracyclines are added next. Oral ***iso*tretinoin** is for severe acne. **Pregnancy tests** are required when using isotretinoin.
Psoriasis	The salmon pink plaques have the **silvery scale of soriasis.** It is worse in winter because summer sunlight helps. Psoriatic **arthritis** is commonly associated.
Stasis dermatitis	The ankle is swollen and red with brown pigment. **The #1 cause of leg ulcers is venous insufficiency** (stasis).

ITCHING

Cause of Itching	*Identification and Important Facts*
Contact dermatitis	Contact leads to itchy erythema on exposed skin. There may be vesicles. Treat with topical steroids.
Atopic dermatitis	Chronic itching starts in infancy or childhood. The reaction is **IgE mediated.** The parents or kid often have hay fever or asthma.
Scabies	The itching is intense with short **burrow lines** in web spaces and skin folds. Treat with lindane lotion and wash sheets and clothes.

CANCER

Neoplasm	*Identification and Important Facts*
Melanoma	Melanomas typically appear as blue or black "moles" with irregular borders and coloring. Depth of invasion predicts survival best.

Neoplasm	*Identification and Important Facts*
Dysplastic nevus	These atypical moles can lead to melanoma. Use total skin photos to follow them. Biopsy anything suspicious.
Basal cell CA*	These firm round nodules or ulcers usually have a **pearly border.** Basal cell carcinoma is **the #1 skin cancer.**
Squamous cell CA*	These firm plaques or nodules typically have a thick scale with no pearly border.
Actinic keratoses*	These rough, scaly, flesh-colored bumps are caused by sun exposure, so they appear on the **face, forearms, and backs of hands.** Freeze them to prevent transformation into squamous cell carcinoma.

* Sun exposure is the #1 risk factor for basal cell carcinoma, squamous cell carcinoma, and actinic keratoses. Caucasians who burn easily are most at risk.

INFECTIONS

Infection	*Identification and Important Facts*
Tinea corporis	Ringworm presents as a red plaque with a **sharp edge and scaly border,** often with central clearing. Do a **KOH prep** on scrapings for fungal hyphae.
Impetigo	The **honey-colored crusts** of impetigo are usually seen on kids. Treat with oral antibiotics that cover Group A *Strep* and *Staph aureus,* such as cephalexin (Keflex).
Hidradenitis suppurativa	The **apocrine glands** are plugged, so inflammation occurs in the axillae or groin. Use antibiotics.

Pityriasis rosea	Macules and papules appear in a **Christmas tree distribution** on the back (''pi**tree**-iasis rosea''). A larger patch precedes the general eruption. It is presumed infectious.

Ophthalmology

- A surprising number of ophthalmology questions may appear on the exam. Most are in the glossy book. Whenever you are presented with a fundus, ask if papilledema is present. With papilledema, the optic disc is severely distorted such that its border is hard to identify.

PAINFUL SEVERE VISION LOSS

- Optic neuritis causes rapid painful vision loss in one eye. Usually **the eye hurts with movement.** Papilledema with these symptoms is diagnostic, but papilledema is not always present. **Multiple sclerosis** is the #1 cause.
- Acute glaucoma causes the sudden onset of severely blurred vision in one eye followed by **excruciating pain.** It is differentiated from optic neuritis by a high intraocular pressure. Acute glaucoma does not cause papilledema.

PAINLESS SEVERE VISION LOSS

- Central retinal artery occlusion causes **sudden painless loss of all vision in one eye.** If it resolves in a few minutes, it is called amaurosis fugax. The retina will be pale with a **cherry-red spot** at the macula. Eye massage can sometimes save the patient's vision. **Temporal arteritis** must be ruled out.
- A cataract is an opacified lens. Cataracts develop over months to years.

PAPILLEDEMA WITH NO VISION CHANGES

- Pseudotumor cerebri (benign intracranial hypertension) is raised intracranial pressure with normal radiologic findings and normal CSF that is under high pressure. **Gross papilledema** is the hallmark. Patients are usually **young overweight women.**
- Increased intracranial pressure with *abnormal* radiologic or CSF findings is an emergency. Tumor, intracranial bleeding, and infection are important causes.

BLURRED VISION WITH CLEAR EYE

- Retinal detachment is **painless.** Vision loss can be minimal or catastrophic, depending on where the retina detaches. The detached portion of the retina looks like a gray cloud.

BLURRED VISION WITH RED EYE

- Anterior uveitis causes **pain, photophobia, and redness** with blurry vision.
- Keratitis is inflammation or ulceration of the cornea. **Pain, photophobia, redness,** and blurry vision occur as in anterior uveitis. Additionally, the eye will be tearing. Keratitis is differentiated from anterior uveitis by eye exam. There is no discharge unless conjunctivitis is also present.

RED EYE WITH NORMAL VISION

- Conjunctivitis leads to discharge without pain. Vision may be blurry due to debris but will clear with blinking.

Abbreviations

AAA	abdominal aortic aneurysm
ABG	arterial blood gas
ACE	angiotensin converting enzyme
ACTH	adrenocorticotropic hormone
ADH	antidiuretic hormone
ADHD	attention deficit hyperactivity disorder
AIDS	acquired immune deficiency syndome
ALL	acute lymphoblastic leukemia
ALT	alanine aminotransferase
AML	acute myeloblastic leukemia
ASD	atrial septal defect
AST	aspartate aminotransferase
AV	atrioventricular
AVSD	atrioventricular septal defect
AZT	zidovudine
β-blockers	beta-blockers
β-HCG	beta-human chorionic gonadotropin
BP	blood pressure
BUN	blood urea nitrogen
C4	fourth cervical vertebra
C5	fifth cervical vertebra
C6	sixth cervical vertebra
CHF	congestive heart failure
CIN	cervical intraepithelial neoplasia
CN V_2	cranial nerve V_2
CN VIII	eighth cranial nerve
CNS	central nervous system
CO	cardiac output
COPD	chronic obstructive pulmonary disease
CPK	creatine phosphokinase
CSF	cerebrospinal fluid
CT	computerized tomogram

ddI	didanosine
DIC	disseminated intravascular coagulation
DNR	do not resuscitate
DSM IV	Diagnostic Standards Manual for Psychiatry, 4th edition
DTs	delirium tremens
DTaP	diphtheria, tetanus, attenuated pertussis
DTP	diphtheria, tetanus, pertussis
ECG	electrocardiogram
ECT	electroconvulsive therapy
ESR	erythrocyte sedimentation rate
FEV_1	forced expiratory volume in 1 second
FHR-UC	fetal heart rate and uterine contraction
FIO_2	fraction of inspired oxygen
FTI	free thyroxine index
FVC	forced vital capacity
GFR	glomerular filtration rate
GI	gastrointestinal
GU	genitourinary
H_2-blockers	histamine type 2 receptor blockers
HCO_3^-	bicarbonate
HDL	high-density lipoprotein
HELLP	hemolytic anemia, elevated liver enzymes, low platelet count
Hib	Hemophilus influenzae type B
HIV	human immunodeficiency virus
HMG-CoA	β-hydroxy-β-methylglutaryl-CoA
HTN	hypertension
Ig	immunoglobulin
IM	intramuscular
ITP	idiopathic thrombocytopenic purpura
IUD	intrauterine device
IUGR	intrauterine growth retardation
IV	intravenous
K^+	potassium
KOH	potassium hydroxide
L5	fifth lumbar vertebra
LDL	low density lipoprotein
LUQ	left upper quadrant
MAO-I	monoamine oxidase inhibitor

MCV	mean corpuscular volume
MEN	multiple endocrine neoplasia
MMR	measles, mumps, rubella
MRI	magnetic resonance imaging
Na^+	sodium
NHL	non-Hodgkin's lymphoma
NSAID	nonsteroidal antiinflammatory drug
NST	nonstress test
ODD	oppositional defiant disorder
OPV	oral polio vaccine
PAN	polyarteritis nodosa
P_{CO_2}	partial pressure of carbon dioxide
PCP	phencyclidine
PCWP	pulmonary capillary wedge pressure
PDA	patent ductus arteriosus
PEEP	positive end expiratory pressure
PKU	phenylketonuria
P_{O_2}	partial pressure of oxygen
PPD	purified protein derivative (test for tuberculosis)
PROM	premature rupture of membranes
PT	prothrombin time
PTT	activated partial thromboplastin time
PVR	peripheral vascular resistance
q	every
RDS	respiratory distress syndrome
RLQ	right lower quadrant
RSV	respiratory syncytial virus
S1	first sacral vertebrae
SaO_2	systemic arterial oxygen saturation
SIADH	syndrome of inappropriate secretion of antidiuretic hormone
SIDS	sudden infant death syndrome
SPEP	serum protein electrophoresis
SSRI	selective serotonin reuptake inhibitor
STD	sexually transmitted disease
SvO_2	systemic venous oxygen saturation
T3	triiodothyronine
T4	thyroxine
TCA	tricyclic antidepressant

TIA	transient ischemic attack
TIBC	total iron binding capacity
TSH	thyroid stimulating hormone
URI	upper respiratory infection
US	United States
USMLE	United States Medical Licensing Exam
UTI	urinary tract infection
VMA	vanillylmandelic acid
VSD	ventricular septal defect

Index

Page numbers followed by *f* indicate figures.

G

H

I

R

S

T

U

V

W

X

Y

Z

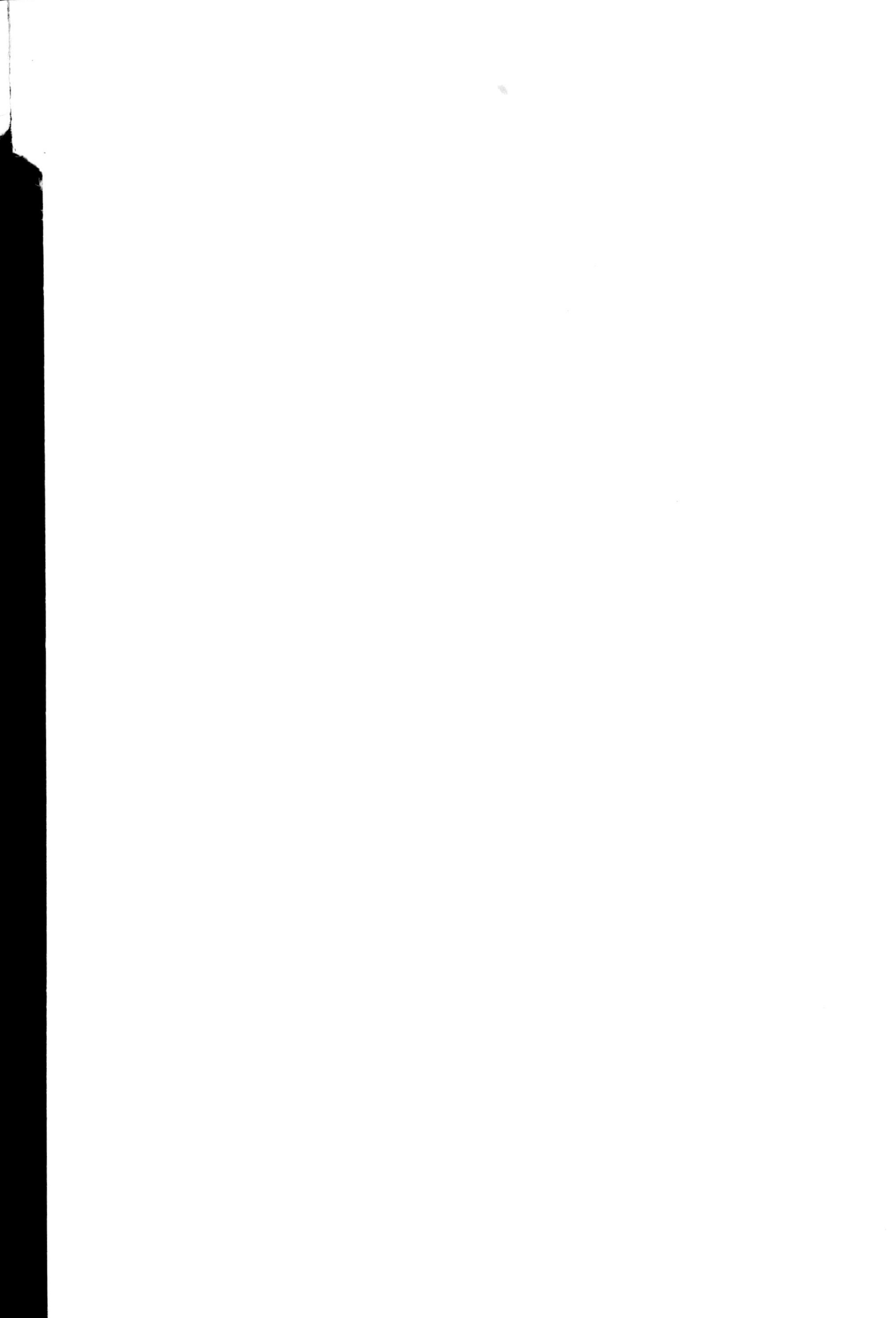

Chemotherapy Drugs

Actinomycin D (Dactinomycin) - inhibits DNA, RNA & protein synthesis (intercalating agent)

Adriamycin (Doxorubicin) - inhibits topoisomerase II & free radical production
- cardiotoxic - usually CHF but may be arrhythmias, peri/myocarditis)

Vincristine - binds to mitotic spindle → metaphase arrest

Vinblastine - inhibits microtubule formation ↑

Bleomycin - inhibits DNA synthesis
pulmonary toxicity - pulmonary fibrosis

Cyclophosphamide - Alkylating Agent
Hemorrhagic cystitis